ideals®
SPRINGTIME

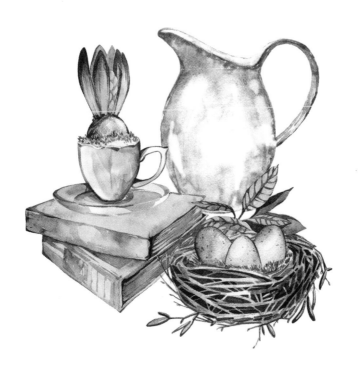

Golden sunshine, a world of green,
a world of blossoms, a breeze so clean;
the redbirds whistle, the bluebirds sing,
my heart rejoices: 'tis spring, 'tis spring!

—CAROLINE HENNING BAIR

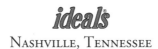
NASHVILLE, TENNESSEE

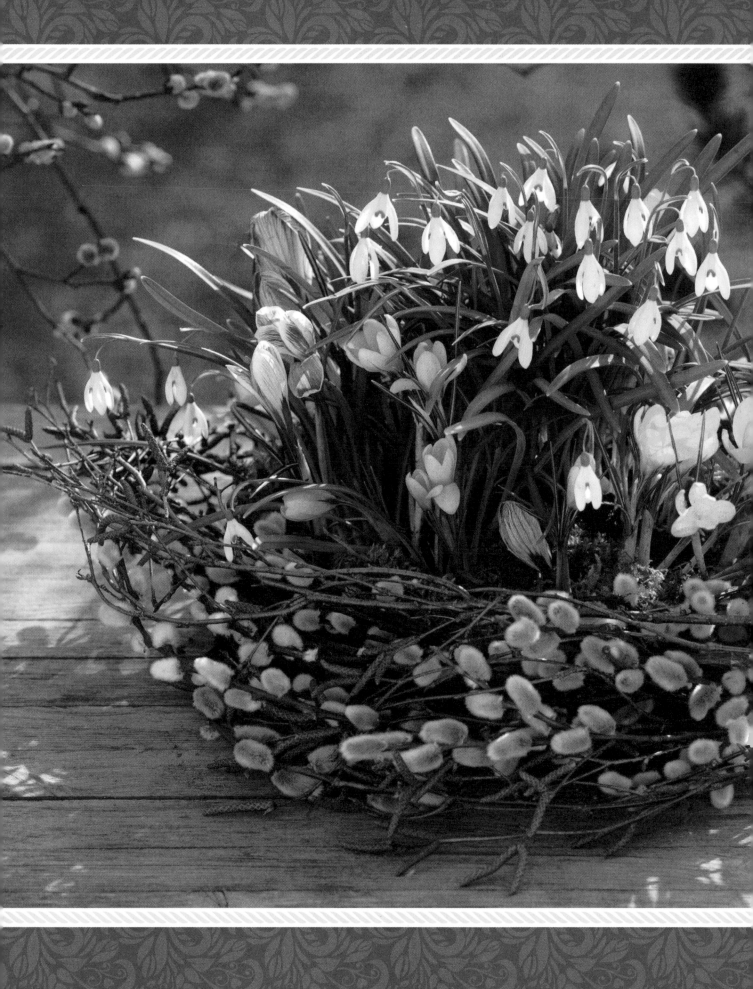

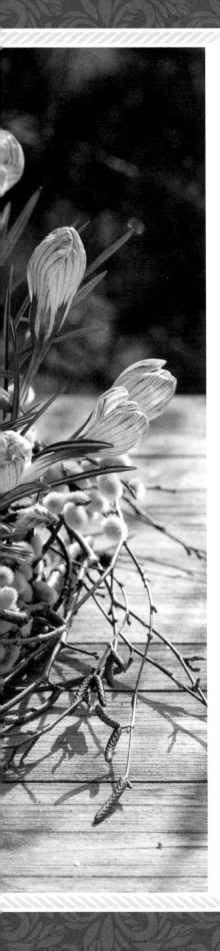

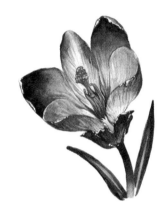

The Coming of Spring
Nora Perry

There's something in the air
that's new and sweet and rare—
a scent of summer things,
a whir as if of wings.

There's something, too,
that's new
in the color of the blue
that's in the morning sky,
before the sun is high.

And though, on plain and hill,
'tis winter, winter still,
there's something seems to say
that winter's had its day.

And all this changing tint,
this whispering stir, and hint
of bud and bloom and wing,
is the coming of the spring.

And tomorrow or today
the brooks will break away

from their icy, frozen sleep
and run and laugh and leap!

And the next thing—
in the woods—
the catkins in their hoods
of fur and silk will stand,
a sturdy little band.

And the tassels soft and fine
of the hazel will untwine,
and the elder-branches show
their buds against the snow.

So, silently but swift,
above the wintry drift,
the long days gain and gain
until, on hill and plain,

once more and yet once more
returning as before,
we see the bloom of birth
make young again the earth.

Photograph © GAP Photos/Friedrich Strauss

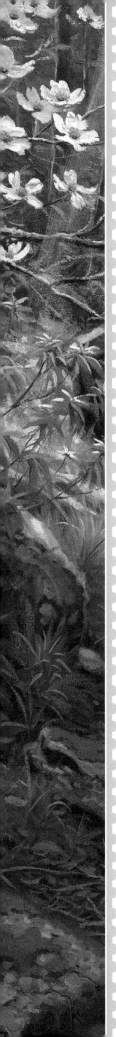
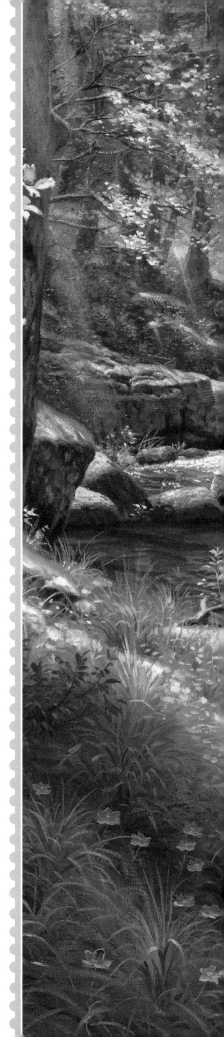

Spring Is Coming
Francis William Bourdillon

By the bursting of the leaves,
by the lengthening of the eves,
spring is coming.
By the flowers that scent the air,
by the skies more blue and fair,
by the singing everywhere,
spring is coming.
All the woods and fields rejoice—
spring is coming.

Early Spring
Rainer Maria Rilke

Harshness vanished. A sudden softness
has replaced the meadows' wintry grey.
Little rivulets of water changed
their singing accents. Tendernesses,
hesitantly, reach toward the earth
from space, and country lanes are showing
these unexpected subtle risings
that find expression in the empty trees.

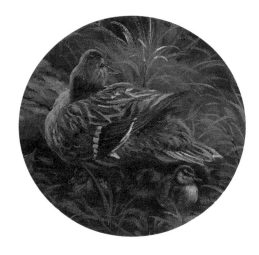

SPRING'S RENEWAL *by Mark Keathley. Image © Mark Keathley*

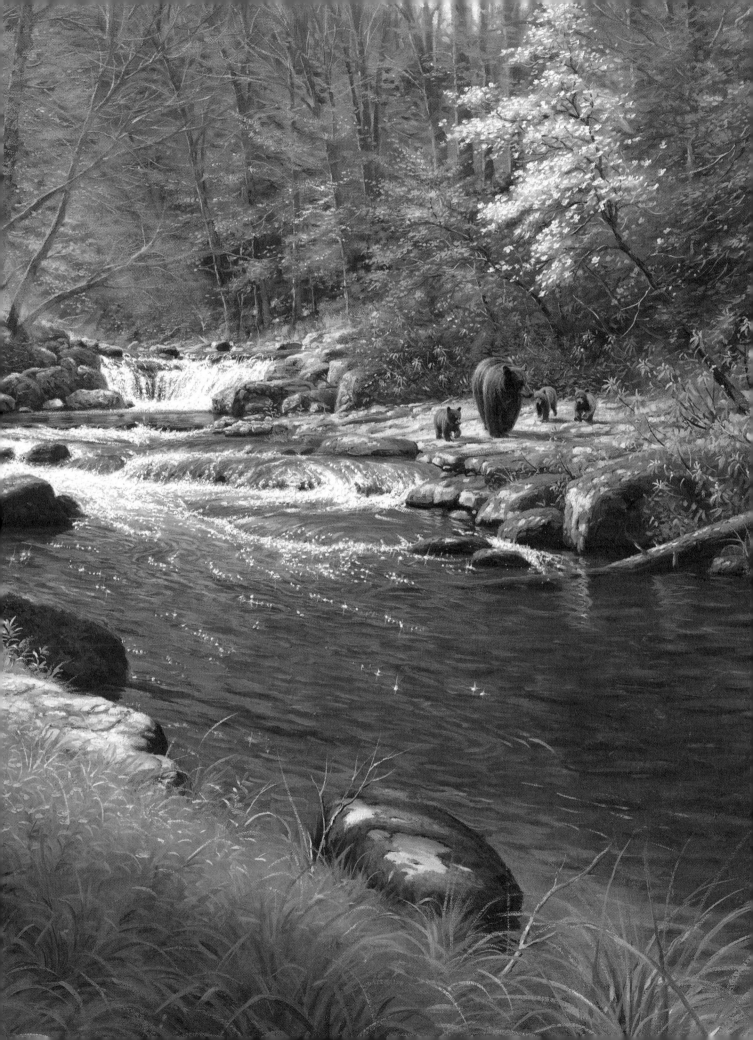

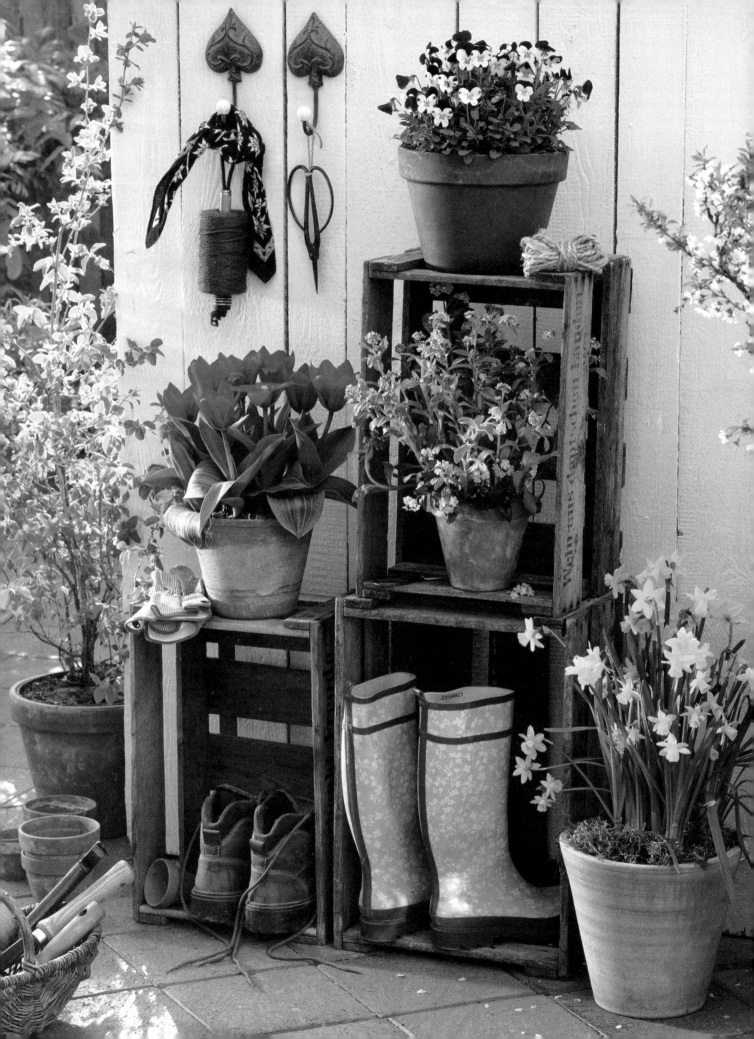

Spring Is in My Heart
Garnett Ann Schultz

Spring is in my heart today;
I know no fear or care,
with hyacinths and tulips
and violets blooming there.
The winter-frosted winds
    may blow
as snowflakes tumble down;
and yet the skies are blue
    up there,
and spring is all around.

Spring is in my mind today,
a beauty so sublime.
(A tender crocus smiled at me—
it can't be wintertime!)
I care not that the world
    is cold—
I feel a warmth so real.
A touch of beauty lights my face,
and it is spring ideal.

Spring is in my world today,
what matter, month or date;
no difference that the winds
    blow cold,
my spring shall not be late.
Beyond the windows of my mind
there's beauty to impart.
My world is blooming
    everywhere,
for spring is in my heart.

**The first day of spring is one thing, and the first spring day is another.
The difference between them is sometimes as great as a month.**
—HENRY VAN DYKE

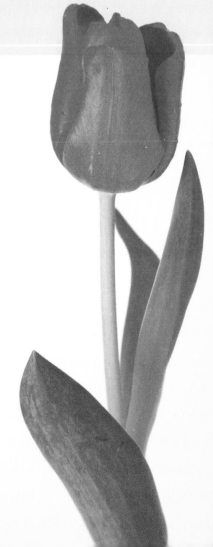

Spring Cleaning
Peggy Mlcuch

Spring cleaning in the garden is
the nicest task of all;
it's sheer delight to wake the plants
I put to sleep last fall.
The tulips and the crocuses
were first to rise, I see;
their green heads down the garden row
are peeking out at me.
The daffodils and hyacinths
are early risers, too,
and soon will join the tulips in
a show of many hues.

Then when I lift the covers from
some other plants, I find
the roses and the peonies
are not too far behind.
The trees are budding all around
and promise that they, too,
will soon burst forth in leafy garb
to brighten up my view.
These tasks I do not view as work;
I cannot wait to start!
Spring cleaning in the garden makes
it springtime in my heart.

Photograph © GAP Photos/Friedrich Strauss

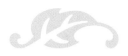

A Burst of Spring

Bea Bourgeois

There is something quietly courageous about a spring garden. These are the survivors: brilliantly colored tulips, daffodils, hyacinths, crocuses, and irises that have slept underground through Mother Nature's cruelest winds and most biting blizzards.

A Midwestern winter is drab and colorless; the piercing white of snow is only occasionally replaced by the sickly brown of a patch of grass showing through melting drifts. We have waited months and months for that first shy burst of splendid color. There is genuine excitement in the cry, "My crocuses are up!" The cycles have repeated; the earth has renewed itself once again.

Even before the snow is all gone, brave spring flowers begin to poke their young green leaves through the cold ground. Then, magically—almost overnight—there are purple, white, yellow, and blazing red hyacinths; glorious yellow daffodils; incredibly hued crimson, pink, yellow, and lavender tulips. The land has come to life, carrying our spirits with it.

More bashful than their city sisters, but no less beautiful, are the delicately colored wildflowers that celebrate springtime. Marsh marigolds poke their bright yellow blossoms through the snow; lavender and white Mayflowers sprout in the woods; the heavy odor of the trailing arbutus is more lovely than an exotic perfume. We begin to understand how badly we have missed seeing color throughout a long and merciless winter. We understand what Wordsworth meant when he compared his lady to "a violet by a mossy stone, half-hidden from the eye; fair as a star, when only one is shining in the sky." If winter comes, can spring indeed be far behind?

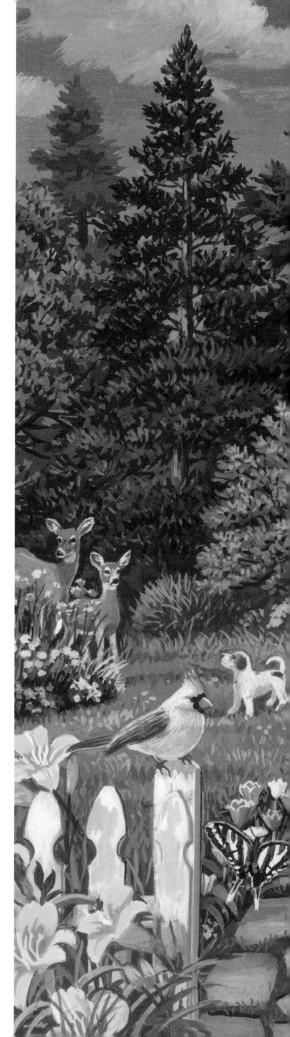

FLOWERS FOR MAMA *by William Vanderdasson.*
Image © William Vanderdasson/Art Licensing

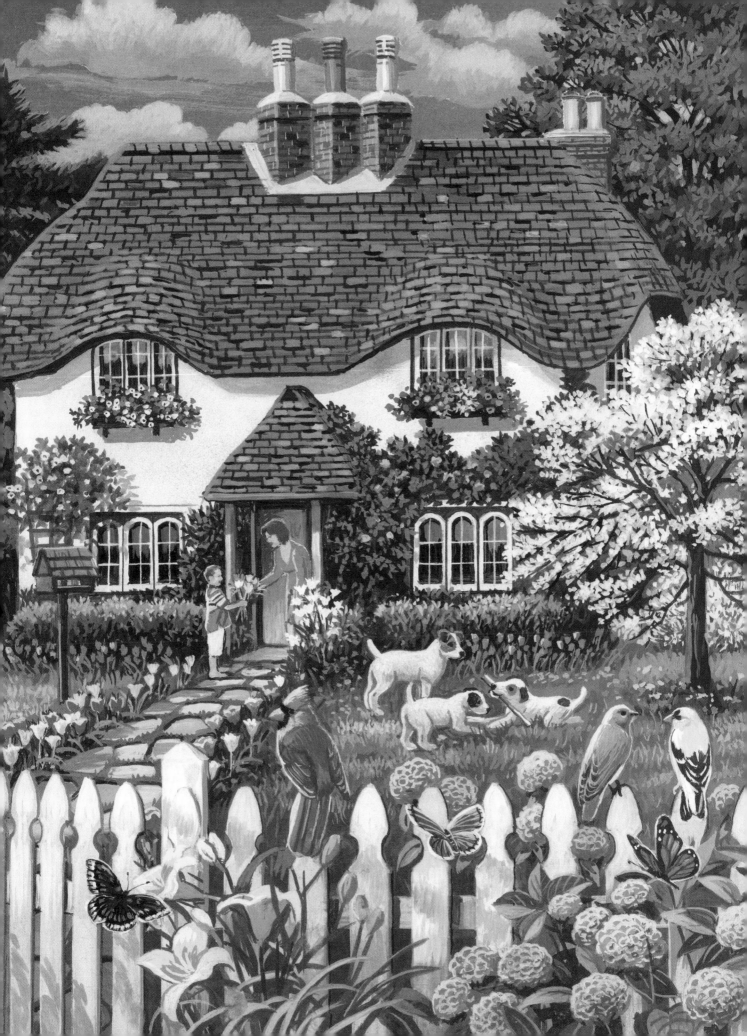

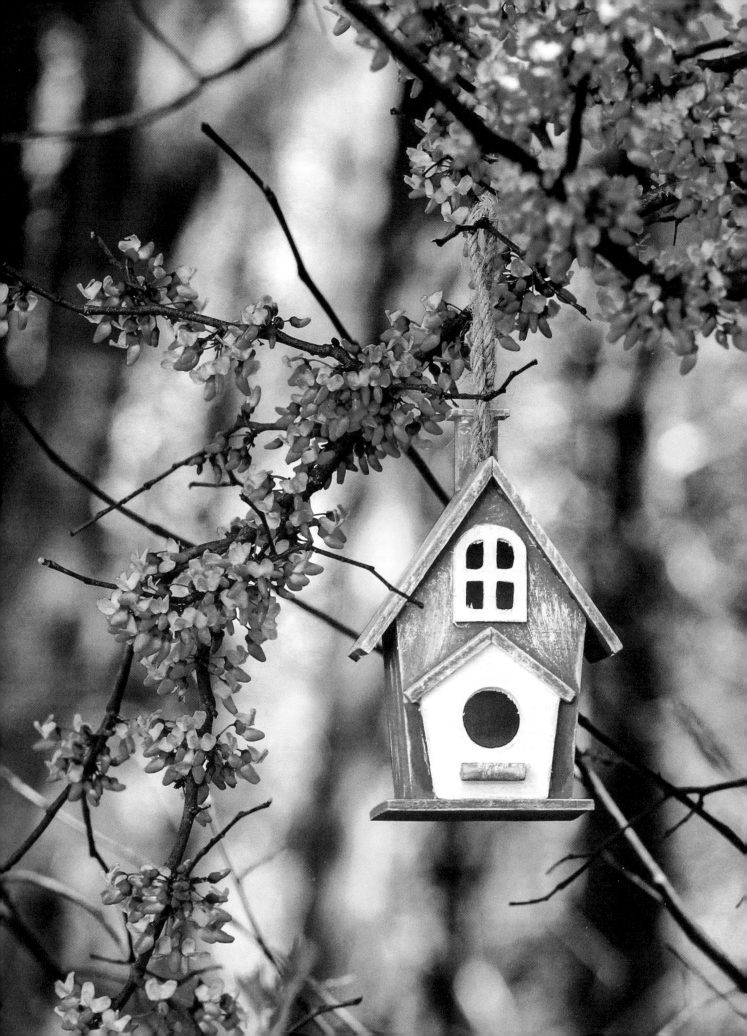

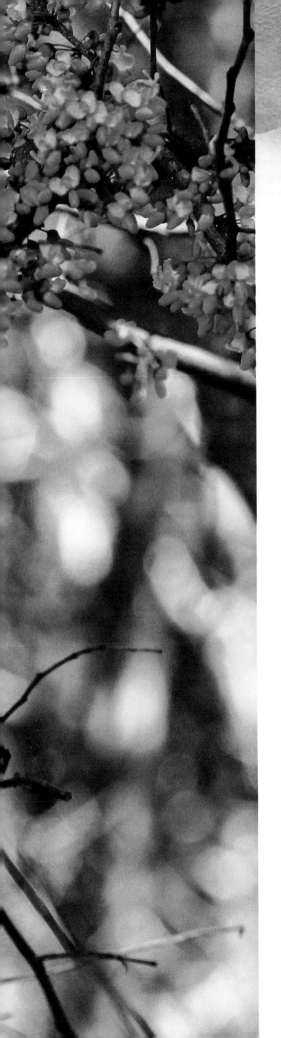

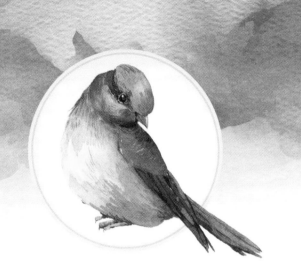

Prayer of a Martha
Eileen Spinelli

Lord, it is spring.
I slip away from
    the lingering
doubts of winter.
I walk through a gate
that needs painting.
Old litter dances underfoot.
I breathe in the scent
of an awakening garden.

I take up brush
and broom
and rusted spade.
There are sweet tasks
to be done.
See—even the
    returning robins
are busy gathering lint
for their nests.

Spring Song
William Griffith

Softly at dawn a whisper stole
down from the green house on the hill,
enchanting many a ghostly hole
and woodsong with the ancient thrill.
Gossiping on the countryside,
spring and wandering breezes say,
God has thrown heaven open wide
and let the thrushes out today.

The Little Plant
Kate L. Brown

In the heart of a seed
buried deep, so deep,
a dear little plant
lay fast asleep.
"Wake!" said the sunshine,
"and creep to the light."
"Wake!" said the voice
of the raindrops bright.
The little plant heard,
and it rose to see
what the wonderful
outside world might be.

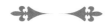

All through
the long winter,
I dream of my garden.
On the first day
of spring, I dig
my fingers deep
into the soft earth.
I can feel its energy,
and my spirits soar.

—HELEN HAYES

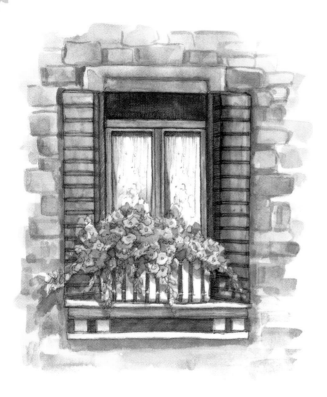

Paint a Rainbow
Agnes Finch Whitacre

Paint me a rainbow,
a rainbow hue,
brush it with lilacs in morning dew;
stroke it with hyacinths and daffodils,
bordering a garden near yonder hills;
on primroses, violas and bleeding hearts
pierced with spears from cupid's darts.
Paint me a rainbow in early spring
and lift it with melodies of birds that sing;
spray it with fragrance of rare perfume
over the gateway to the month of June!

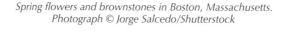

Spring flowers and brownstones in Boston, Massachusetts.
Photograph © Jorge Salcedo/Shutterstock

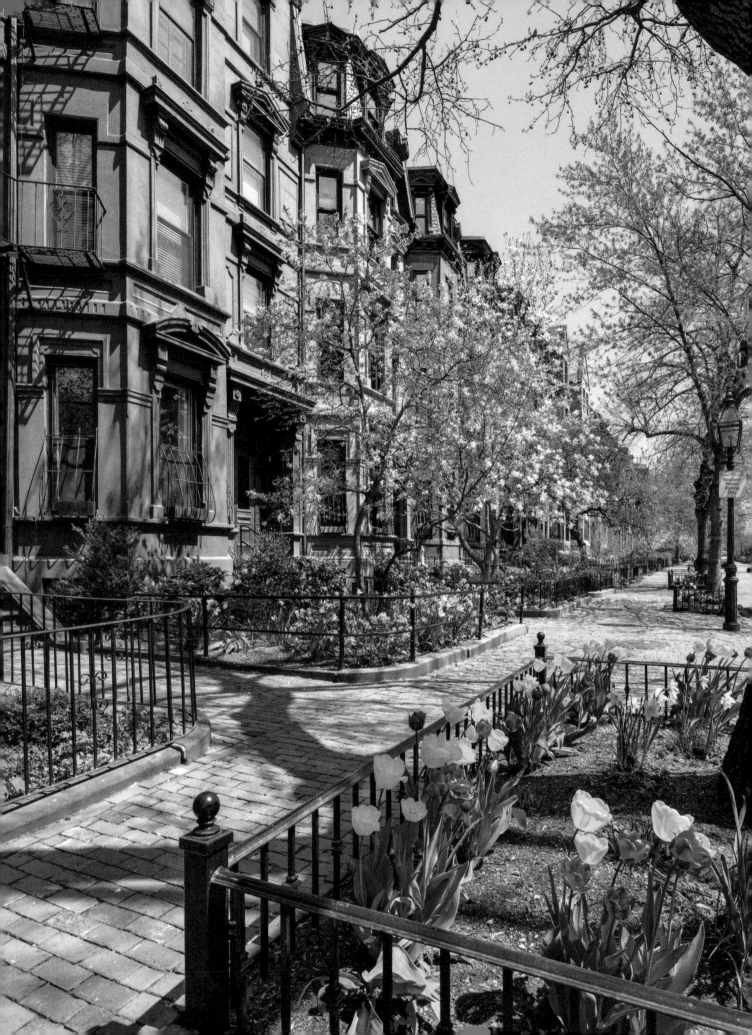

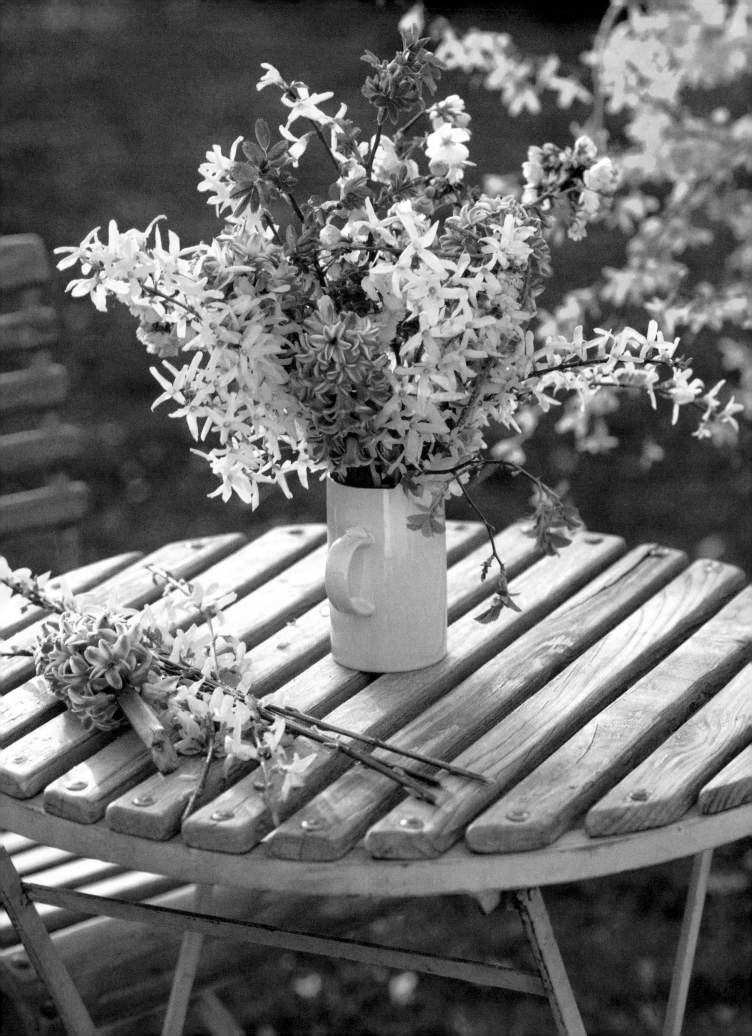

A Light Exists in Spring

Emily Dickinson

A light exists in spring
not present on the year
at any other period.
When March is scarcely
   here

a color stands abroad
on solitary hills
that science cannot
   overtake,
but human nature feels.

It waits upon the lawn;
it shows the furthest tree

upon the furthest slope
   we know;
it almost speaks to me.

Then, as horizons step,
or noons report away,
without the formula of sound,
it passes, and we stay:

a quality of loss
affecting our content,
as trade had suddenly
   encroached
upon a sacrament.

Forsythia

Amanda Meade Brewer

Ah! On branches brown and bare
a thousand yellow butterflies
have settled—swinging—
small wings suspended in the air,
with Midas touch—bringing
gold to April!

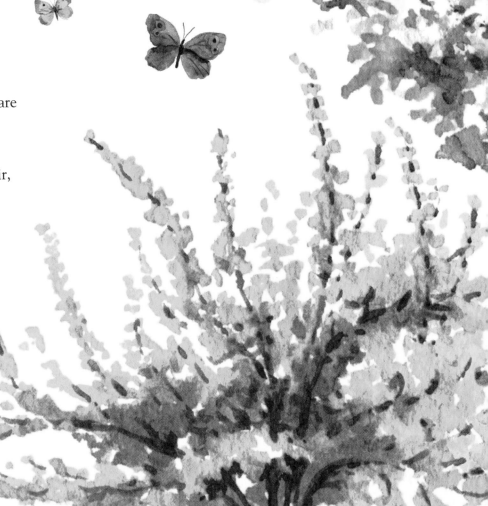

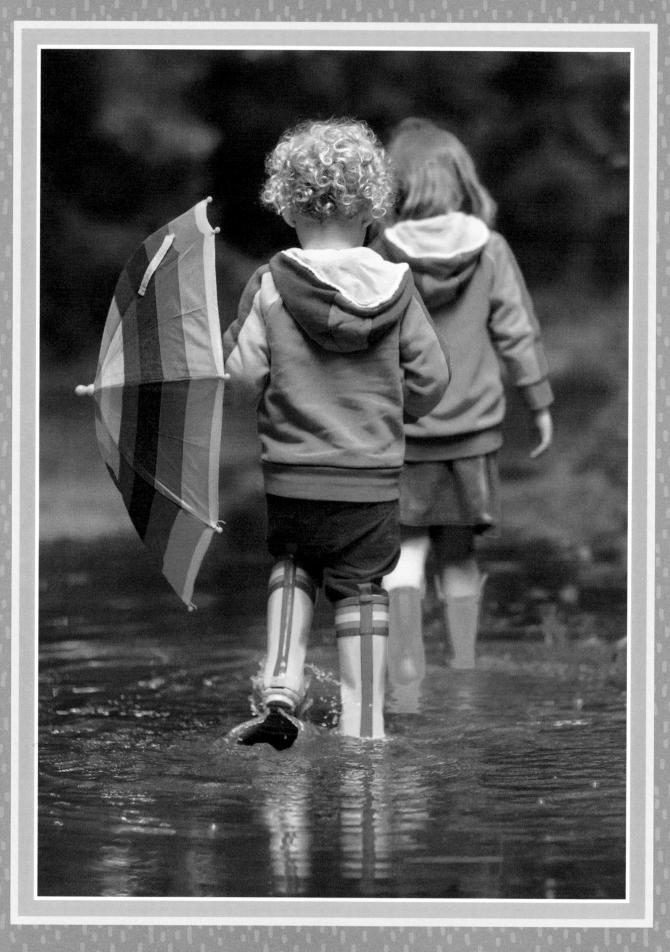

April Rain
Marion Doyle

The April rain
is a little-boy rain:
he scribbles notes
on the windowpane;
he wades the puddles
on skipping feet
and bounces silver balls
in the street.

An Umbrella Day
Minnie Klemme

It is an umbrella day;
there's water in the street,
all the gutters running,
galoshes on our feet.

In the April wetness,
there is a note of cheer:
just a wiff of violets
give promise spring is here.

Rainy Day
Edna Jaques

It isn't just a rainy day,
although the wind is chill;
there is a fragrance blowing down
from every common hill.
A robin with a scarlet vest
is hunting moss to line her nest.

The hedgerows have a tinge of green
like mist above a bog;
a squirrel is scolding like a shrew
from an old cedar log;
a pear tree in a sheltered nook
has taken on a springtime look.

The rain is softening up the earth
with tiny hammer strokes,
bringing new growth to
    meadow grass,
new leaves to ancient oaks.
It's washing all the walks
    and walls,
and making beauty as it falls.

The air is laden with the scent
of fresh earth newly plowed;
the sun is trying hard to break
through a thin piece of cloud
and giving to the countryside
the radiance of a happy bride.

It isn't just a rainy sky.
It's winter bidding earth goodbye.

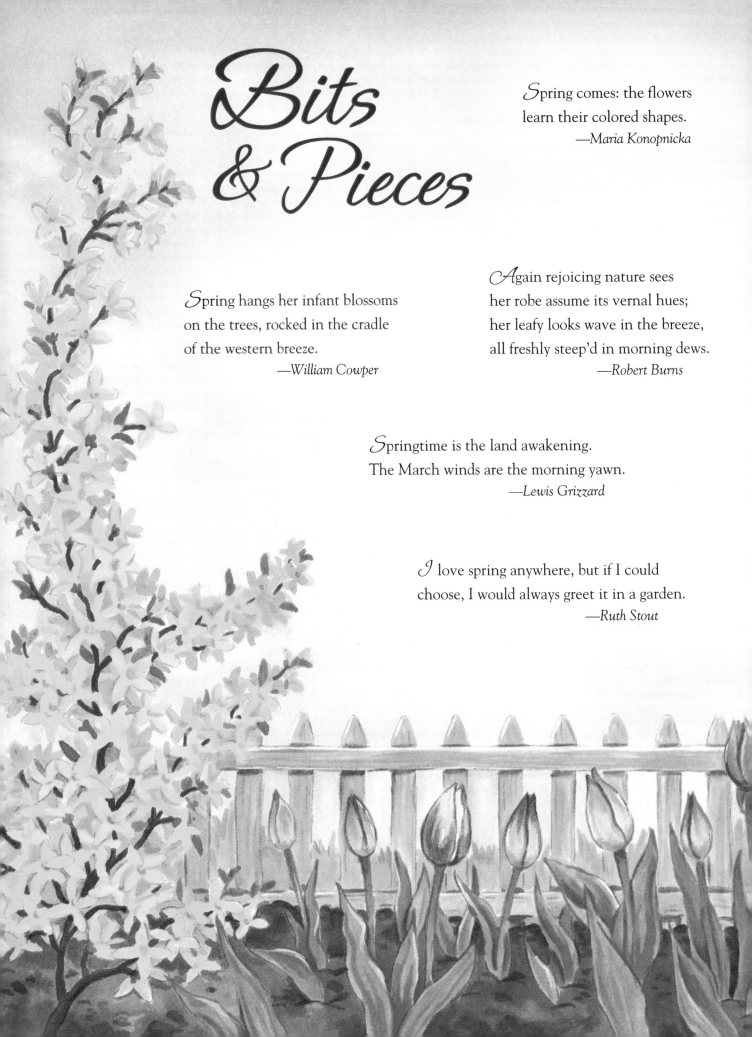

Bits & Pieces

Spring comes: the flowers
learn their colored shapes.
—Maria Konopnicka

Spring hangs her infant blossoms
on the trees, rocked in the cradle
of the western breeze.
—William Cowper

Again rejoicing nature sees
her robe assume its vernal hues;
her leafy looks wave in the breeze,
all freshly steep'd in morning dews.
—Robert Burns

Springtime is the land awakening.
The March winds are the morning yawn.
—Lewis Grizzard

I love spring anywhere, but if I could
choose, I would always greet it in a garden.
—Ruth Stout

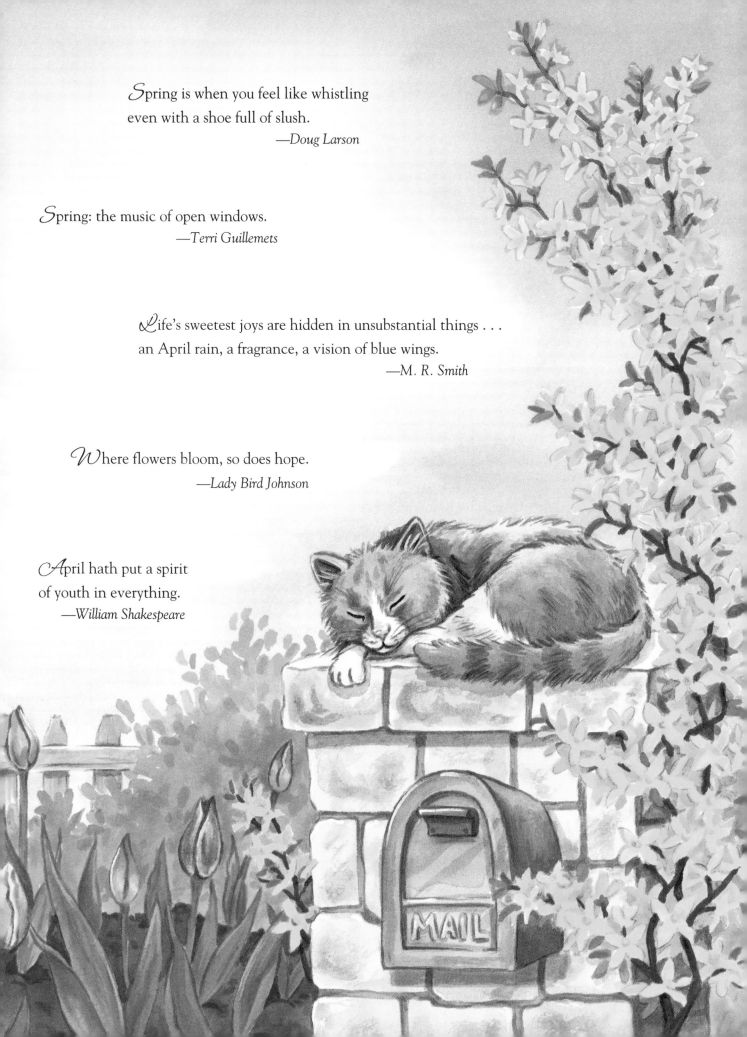

Spring is when you feel like whistling
even with a shoe full of slush.
—Doug Larson

Spring: the music of open windows.
—Terri Guillemets

Life's sweetest joys are hidden in unsubstantial things . . .
an April rain, a fragrance, a vision of blue wings.
—M. R. Smith

Where flowers bloom, so does hope.
—Lady Bird Johnson

April hath put a spirit
of youth in everything.
—William Shakespeare

MAIL

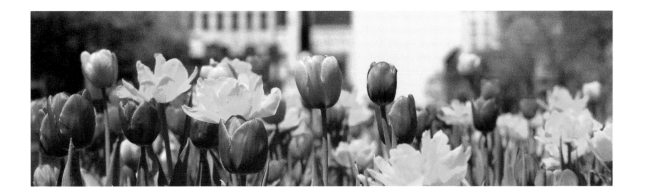

City Spring

Anne Kennedy Brady

Perhaps it is my current locale—Chicago, where winters are famously miserable—but I love spring in the city. I have nothing against expansive fields of rural tulips or newly hatched ducklings waddling beside a picturesque suburban pond. But my heart sings loudest when I see a brave little crocus push through dingy concrete and watch a robin redbreast perch on first one fire escape railing, then another, then another, before swooping down to select its breakfast from my neighbor's tiny backyard garden.

And then there is the renewed bustle. The moment the temperature stretches above fifty-five degrees, my neighborhood seems to awaken. Faces previously buried in scratchy scarves emerge to greet gentler weather. We look at each other as if to say, "Can you believe this?"—as if we've once again received permission to greet strangers as friends, with warm eyes and easy smiles. No longer do we enter restaurants and cafes hurried and over-grateful, like polar explorers, as the proprietors offer pitying expressions and drippy coat racks. No longer do we see our neighbors only in the stairwells, rushing from heated apartments to heated cars, and back again. Restaurants open their windows. Cafes set up their patio furniture. My upstairs neighbor blasts music from his rooftop deck and invites us up for lemonade. And while sixty degrees isn't quite lemonade weather, we happily accept.

As the mother of a busy toddler, I am especially excited for spring this year. Winter is long for little legs that yearn to run farther than the length of our playroom. We have made the rounds of music classes and toddler yoga, and scoped out the best library story times; but, let's be honest, there's nothing quite like a swing set. Fortunately, we live within walking distance of two large playgrounds (four, when the elementary school across the street lets out for the day). When the sun makes its long-awaited appearance each spring, so do the mommies, daddies, nannies, and their charges, reveling in sandboxes and monkey bars and good, old-fashioned dirt. As our kids learn to share dump trucks and sand shovels, we learn to share our lives with other grown-ups again, and new friendships blossom.

Don't get me wrong: I am not saying that spring in the city is more beautiful than spring anywhere else. If I base my analysis purely on foliage, it's objectively less beautiful than springtime on a flower-splashed countryside. But for me, the promise of spring is most obvious smack-dab in the middle of the urban jungle. Resilience is on full display when a bird builds its nest atop the pillar of an immovable concrete building. When someone boards the train with a bouquet of fresh flowers, and everyone around him looks up from their phones or their newspapers, smiling in spite of their to-do lists. A shared moment of joy and relief. Color amid the gray. Life despite the stone.

The city constantly demands our full attention. We are told to shop at this store, hire this person, finish this project, purchase this strange coffee concoction. But inevitably, and with stubborn grit, spring pushes through the noise. Slivers of sunshine cut the chill and draw our gaze to constant, small surprises. "Here I am!" the crocus seems to say, grinning against a backdrop of cement and commotion. "I made it through the winter! And so did you."

Spring Rhubarb Lemonade

5	cups chopped rhubarb	1½	cups freshly squeezed lemon juice
¾	cup granulated sugar	2	cups lemon-lime soda
1	tablespoon grated lemon zest		

In a saucepan, stir together 3½ cups water, rhubarb, sugar, and lemon zest. Bring to a boil, stirring until sugar is dissolved. Reduce heat, cover, and simmer 20 minutes. Let the rhubarb mixture cool, then pour through a wire-mesh strainer set over a large pitcher. Press on solids to extract as much liquid as possible. Discard solids. Stir in lemon juice and soda. Serve over ice, garnished with a sprig of mint. Makes 6 servings.

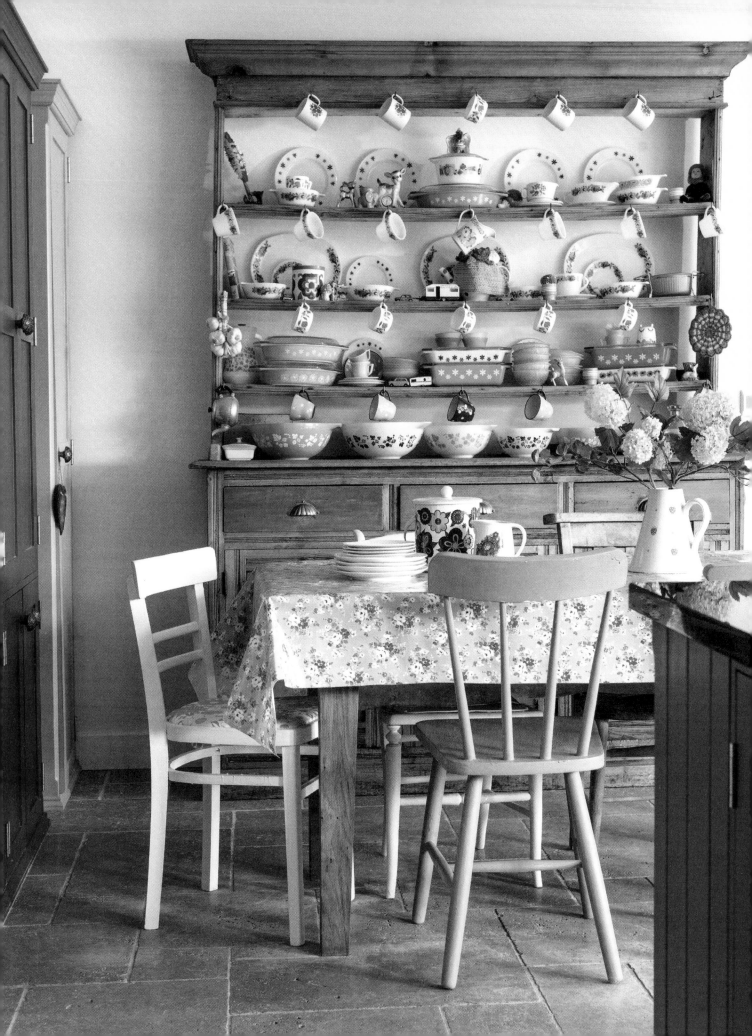

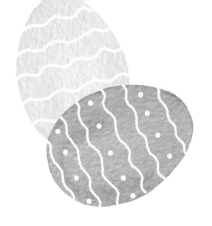

Memory
Shirley Sallay

Eastertime means Easter eggs
of rainbow-colored hue;
a soft and cuddly bunny
and a jellybean or two;
a brand-new Easter bonnet
on top of baby's head;
a bit of artificial grass
in green, or gold, or red;

a little woven basket
beside each bedroom door,
where children may discover them
at dawn, as they explore.

Just a bit of whimsy
    for a special holiday—
moments shared together,
then gently tucked away.

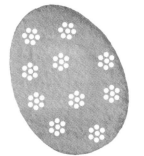

History Repeats
Reginald Holmes

The Easters of our childhood
will always be a part
of those happy recollections
that linger in the heart.

Mother dyed the Easter eggs
when we had gone to rest
and called us early in the morn
to find the bunny's nest.

It seems we hunted everywhere
and let our breakfast wait;

we looked behind the evergreens
close by the garden gate.

But underneath the lilac bush,
at last, our eyes would view
a lovely little nest of eggs
of yellow, pink, and blue.

But history does repeat itself,
when all the years have flown . . .
now we are hiding Easter eggs
for children of our own!

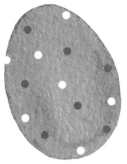

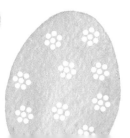

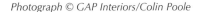

The Easter Egg

Andrew L. Luna

One Saturday years ago, I was starting my annual spring yard work. It was a couple of weeks before Easter, and the seasonal color was beginning to emerge. While I was trimming grass and weeds close to the house, I noticed something odd. I parted the tall grass around one of our shrubs and recognized an Easter egg from the previous year, apparently never found.

I pulled the purple plastic egg out of the grass. It was faded and dirty from sitting outside for almost a year, and it rattled when I shook it. I opened it to reveal the misshapen remains of what used to be a piece of candy. Taking a break from my work, I sat in a chair in the shade of a tree. I looked at the egg, turning it over and over in my hand, and a flood of Easter memories came to my mind.

What I held in my hand represented the original Easter egg hunt, nearly a year before, for our then-3-year-old twins, Jay and Jessica. I remembered that day fondly. It had been a Saturday, the day before Easter, and I had the important job of hiding the eggs while my wife kept our twins busy in the house and prepared their straw baskets with multi-colored Easter grass.

I quickly hid the eggs in places that would not be too difficult for a three-year-old to find. While doing so, I realized that I was having as much fun hiding them as my twins would have finding them. When I opened the front door to let everyone know the hunt was ready to begin, the twins burst excitedly out of the house. They knew that there was a piece of candy in each egg—except one special egg that held a dollar bill.

Jay and Jessica searched eagerly, looking beside rocks, in the mailbox, under bushes and up in trees for the colored treasure. Jay even made a point of looking exactly where his sister looked, in hopes of finding something she had missed. Seeing our twins running around the yard laughing and having a good time, my mind drifted back to my childhood days and how Mom always bought Easter egg dye to color our freshly boiled eggs. While I never really liked the smell of the vinegar and water solution, I

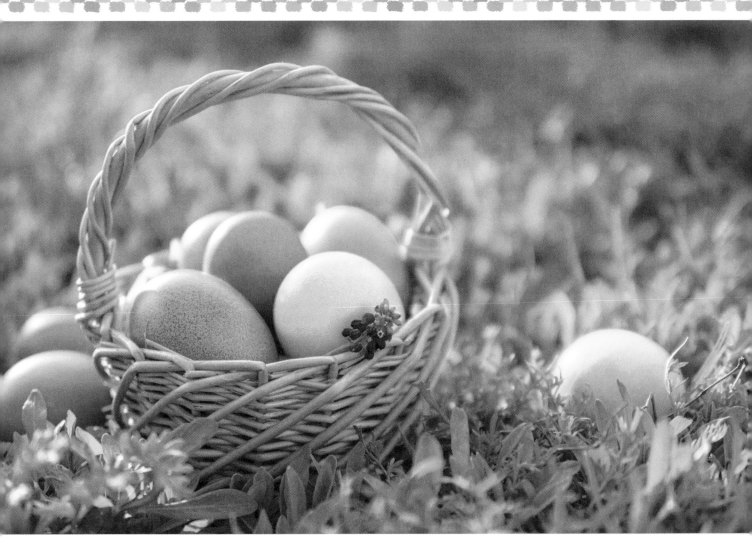

loved the rich, spring colors that seemed to magically affix to the eggs once they were immersed in the liquid dye.

A shout for joy snapped me back to the hunt underway—Jessica had found the special golden egg with the dollar inside. She made the decision that she wanted to split her winnings with her brother. (Our twins have always been that way, and we are blessed for it.) Once we thought we had located all the eggs, we went inside for baths, dinner, and bed. It was a great day.

As I continued to hold in my hand the plastic egg from that first hunt a year before, I got up from my chair and looked around for new places to hide this year's treasure. I smiled, knowing this old egg symbolized a treasured new tradition—of hiding and hunting Easter eggs with our twins.

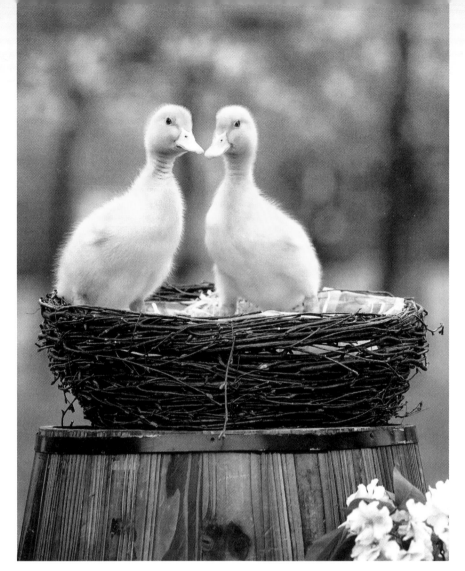

A Fine-Feathered Easter

Cindy La Ferle

When you really think about it, Americans do strange things to celebrate religious holidays.

Consider Easter. There's nothing particularly pious about hiding neon pink and blue plastic eggs in the backyard. And it's not exactly Christian to give someone a milk-chocolate rabbit, especially if the recipient is on a diet.

Even more bewildering was the pair of live ducklings my uncle gave me for Easter when I was a child. I don't recall the looks on my parents' faces when my uncle handed me the cardboard box containing two fuzzy ducklings peeping at the tops of their tiny lungs. But I remember being told right away that I couldn't keep them both.

A neighborhood playmate agreed to adopt one of the ducklings. After a couple of weeks the poor thing was sent to a relative's farm up north, where it became a holiday dinner entree the following spring. For lack of a better idea, my parents bought a small swimming pool and reluctantly allowed me to keep my duckling in our backyard.

Like most suburbanites, my mom and dad were totally clueless about farm animals, so our new pet initially stirred up some gender confusion. As the weeks passed, the duck I had named Oliver matured and sprouted a mass of dazzling white feathers. Raised in rural Scotland, my grandfather knew immediately that Oliver was really an Olivia.

"A male duck has a curl at the end of his tail," Grandpa said. "The females have a plain tail like Oliver's." It wasn't long before Grandpa was proven right. One morning, Oliver left a large egg in the small shed where she slept—and from then on, we found a fresh egg in her bedding every day.

Of course, it took the neighbors awhile to get used to our exceptional pet. Some were startled when they heard Oliver's daily wake-up quack around seven a.m. And Mrs. Ritchie, who lived on the street behind us, says she still remembers watching the duck waddle next to me whenever I visited my friends around the block.

Oliver was no birdbrain. She never let me out of her sight when she was away from home. But as soon as she recognized our house, she'd hightail it back to her blue plastic swimming pool in the backyard.

She was also sharp enough to understand it was feeding time whenever she heard the sound of a spoon banging on the side of a dish. Her diet consisted mostly of dried corn from a nearby feed store or a plate of finely chopped hard-boiled eggs. For dessert she enjoyed the pansies in my mother's garden.

If her wake-up quack didn't produce the desired result, Oliver would nibble at the screen on my bedroom window in the morning. When I appeared outside, she would bow and stretch her long neck in greeting, which always thrilled me.

In retrospect, Oliver wasn't the easiest pet to care for, and I wouldn't recommend keeping a duck for a pet in the suburbs. Backyard captivity isn't fair to any creature that ordinarily thrives in a rural setting.

At the end of Oliver's second summer with us, we returned from a family vacation to discover she had died in our backyard. The neighbor who was caring for her could only guess that she'd been attacked by a predatory animal.

Oliver's stay with us was brief but eventful, and it sparked my near-religious devotion to birds and animals. Years later, I can't think of Easter without remembering her.

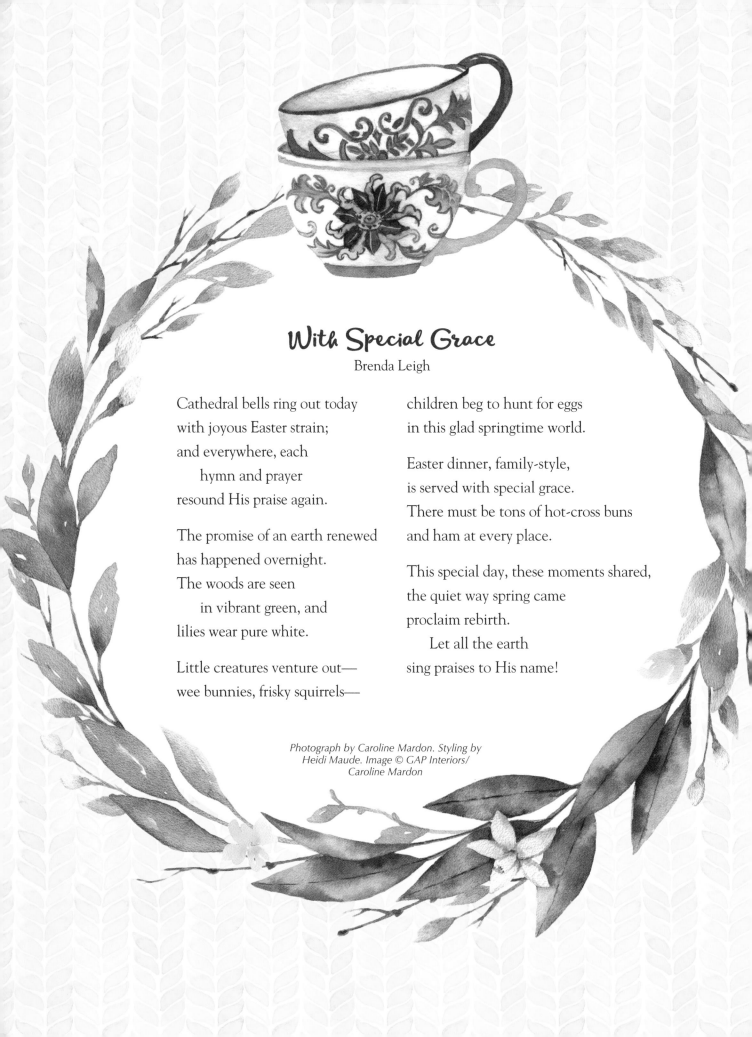

With Special Grace

Brenda Leigh

Cathedral bells ring out today
with joyous Easter strain;
and everywhere, each
    hymn and prayer
resound His praise again.

The promise of an earth renewed
has happened overnight.
The woods are seen
    in vibrant green, and
lilies wear pure white.

Little creatures venture out—
wee bunnies, frisky squirrels—

children beg to hunt for eggs
in this glad springtime world.

Easter dinner, family-style,
is served with special grace.
There must be tons of hot-cross buns
and ham at every place.

This special day, these moments shared,
the quiet way spring came
proclaim rebirth.
    Let all the earth
sing praises to His name!

*Photograph by Caroline Mardon. Styling by
Heidi Maude. Image © GAP Interiors/
Caroline Mardon*

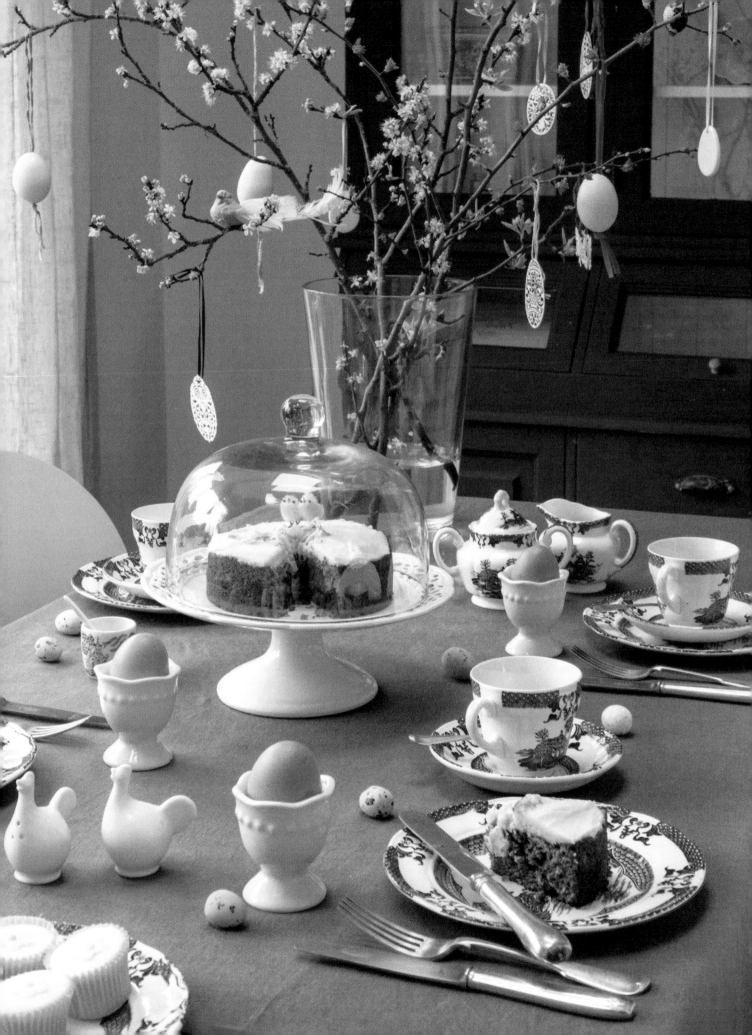

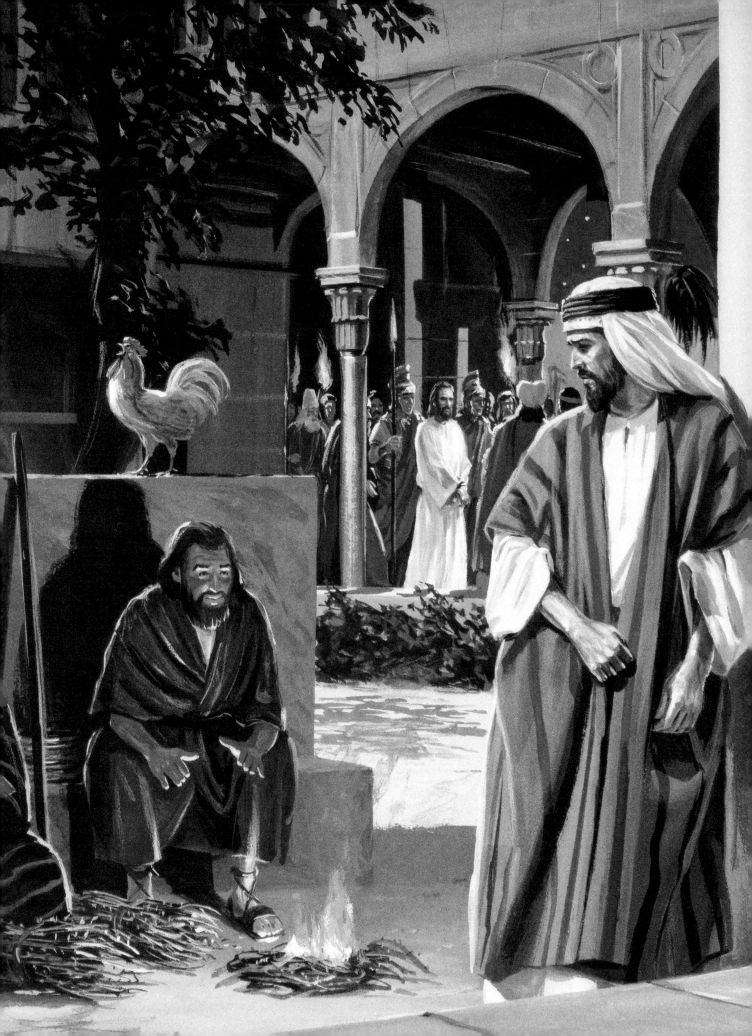

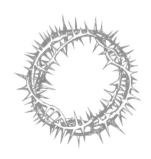

The Denial
B. Muenta

Urged, Lord, by sinful terror,
Peter denied Thy name.
Soon, conscious of his error,
he mourned his guilt with shame.
Thy look with sorrow filled his breast;
he sought Thy pard'ning mercy
and was with pardon blessed.

After, how grew this martyr
in faith and hardihood!
He scorned Thy truth to barter,
but sealed it with his blood:
for Thee, his Lord, he spent his breath,
in life declared Thy glory,
and honored Thee in death.

The Meaning of the Look
Elizabeth Barrett Browning

I think that look of Christ might seem to say—
"Thou Peter! art thou then a common stone
which I at last must break My heart upon
for all God's charge to His high angels may
guard My foot better? Did I yesterday
wash thy feet, My beloved, that they should run
quick to deny Me 'neath the morning sun?
And do thy kisses, like the rest, betray?
The cock crows coldly. Go, and manifest
a late contrition, but no bootless fear!
For when thy final need is dreariest,
thou shalt not be denied, as I am here;
My voice to God and angels shall attest,
Because I know this man, let him be clear."

Good Friday
Christina Rossetti

Am I a stone, and not a sheep,
that I can stand, O Christ, beneath Thy cross,
to number drop by drop Thy blood's slow loss,
and yet not weep?
Not so those women loved
who with exceeding grief lamented Thee;
not so fallen Peter weeping bitterly;
not so the thief was moved;
not so the Sun and Moon
which hid their faces in a starless sky,
a horror of great darkness at broad noon—
I, only I. Yet give not o'er,
but seek Thy sheep, true Shepherd
    of the flock;
greater than Moses, turn and look once more
and smite a rock.

Peter's Story

Dr. Ralph F. Wilson

By day it gnawed at him, but nights were even worse. He had betrayed his dearest friend. Not privately, not secretly, but blatantly, out in the open for all the world to see. And now it was too late to say, "I'm sorry." His friend was dead.

Peter tossed sleeplessly, unable to find a position that felt comfortable. Outside, he could hear the sounds of Jerusalem stirring to life. This city he had once loved to visit, he now hated. It held too many painful memories impossible to erase from his mind. Today he would leave for Galilee and fishing, though even fishing held no allure for him now. Nothing did.

For the thousandth time he cursed himself. "He was my friend! How could I have done this to my very best friend?"

He could see Jesus riding that donkey down the hill into Jerusalem to the cheers of thousands. He saw Him in hot anger overturning coin-laden tables in the temple. "You have made My Father's house a den of thieves!" the Master had told them in carefully measured but biting words.

Peter recalled blind men abruptly seeing, lame men suddenly walking, and loathsome lepers' skin turning baby-soft within a moment of Jesus' touch. He saw Jesus' smile, His compassion, His hours of gentle teaching. He felt the Master's hand on his shoulder after a long day of caring for the multitudes. The accompanying words repeated themselves over and over in his mind, *"Thanks, Peter, for your help today. You are a faithful friend . . .*

a faithful friend . . . a faithful friend." Tears began to well up in Peter's eyes. *Faithful? Me?*

When the high priest's soldiers had tried to arrest Jesus, Peter had defended his Master with a sword. But later, when a servant girl had challenged him with: "You're one of His disciples, aren't you?" he had denied it with an oath.

A mere servant girl! But again and again he had compounded the cowardly lie until the cock crowed, and Jesus' eyes from far across the courtyard met his. Sad, disappointed eyes. Then he had broken and run. Run from the high priest's home into the dark streets. Run until he could run no more. Run until he had flung himself onto the cobbled streets sobbing. Later that morning, he had watched from a distance as they mocked and tormented his friend, finally nailing hands and feet with huge spikes, and suspending Him from a cross until His life was spent. He couldn't bear another day in this city!

The thin light of dawn had appeared under the door. Night was finally over; today he would leave. Today he would run away, back to the only life he knew. Today Peter would leave this bloody city behind.

Bang! Bang! The nearby door shook as someone kept banging on it. Peter reached for his sword and quietly took his place behind the door.

"Peter, John, it's Mary! Let me in." It was a woman's voice, Mary Magdalene, one of Jesus' close friends who had traveled with them for

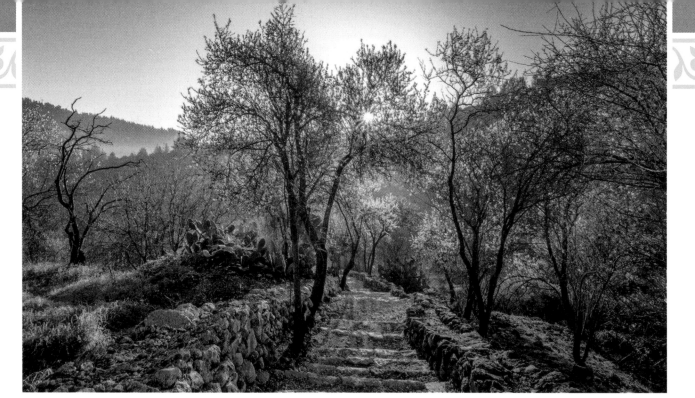

Sunrise through almond trees in Jerusalem Hills, in Israel. Image © John Theodor/Shutterstock

months. He unbolted the door and Mary slipped inside. She took several deep breaths before she could speak, then blurted out her message: "They've stolen the body! Jesus' body is gone, and we don't know where they've put Him!"

John, who was wide awake by now, looked at Peter, and then threw on his clothes. Peter was out the door running, running down the streets, tearing around corners, headed for the garden tomb where Jesus' body had been laid.

Now John was close behind. Younger and faster, John soon outdistanced Peter. By the time Peter got to the tomb, John was standing outside the opening, peering in. The huge stone, designed to prevent desecration of the tomb, was rolled away. Peter brushed inside. It took a moment for his eyes to adjust to the dimness of the damp limestone cave.

There was the linen gravecloth that had been wrapped turn after turn around the body. It lay on the chiseled stone shelf where the body had been. Yet now, with nothing inside, its coils lay collapsed, empty, like a chrysalis after the butterfly has emerged. Folded separately was the cloth that had been around Jesus' head.

Peter looked at John and motioned him inside. How curious! If the tomb had been robbed and the body stolen, he would have expected the wrappings to be nowhere in sight. Or perhaps strewn in haste around the narrow stone room. Yet here they were, orderly, as if laid aside, no longer needed.

John looked at Peter. Peter looked at John. Peter could catch the faintest smile playing at the corners of John's mouth.

What if . . . ? What if . . . He is risen?

Peter walked back into Jerusalem, but each step was a bit quicker than the one before. What if He is risen?

As Peter turned the corner onto the street where he was staying, he saw a figure waiting for him at the door. A very familiar figure—Jesus!

Peter *ran* to meet Him!

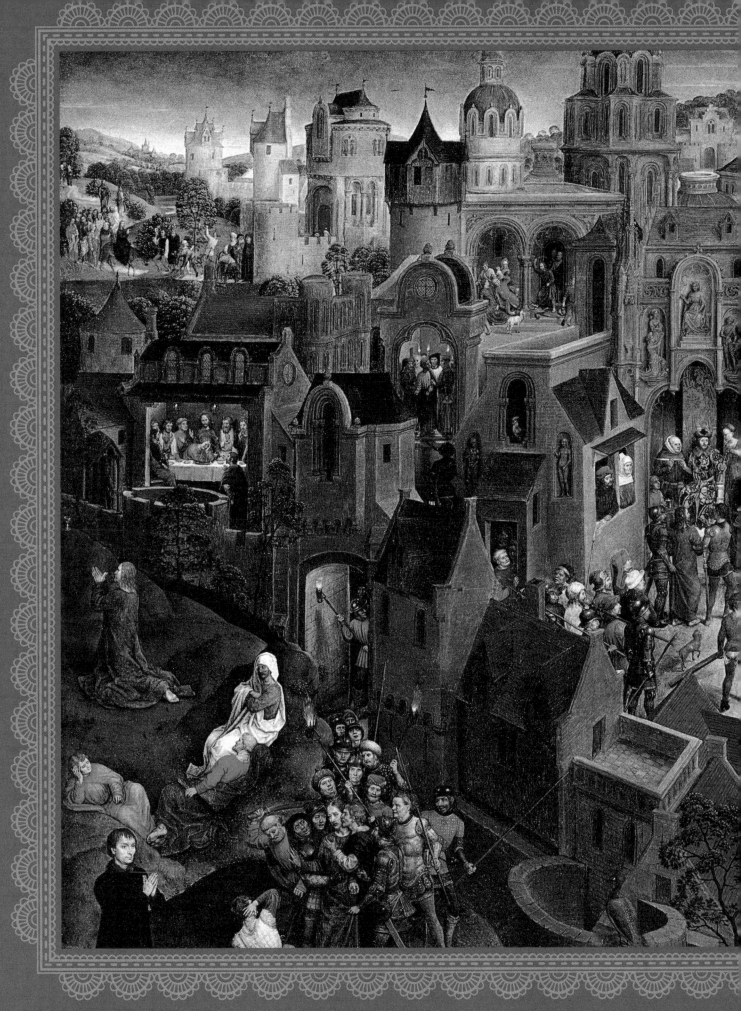

The Last Supper

Luke 22:7–23

Then came the day of unleavened bread, when the passover must be killed. And he sent Peter and John, saying, Go and prepare us the passover, that we may eat. And they said unto him, Where wilt thou that we prepare? And he said unto them, Behold, when ye are entered into the city, there shall a man meet you, bearing a pitcher of water; follow him into the house where he entereth in. And ye shall say unto the goodman of the house, The Master saith unto thee, Where is the guestchamber, where I shall eat the passover with my disciples? And he shall shew you a large upper room furnished: there make ready.

And they went, and found as he had said unto them: and they made ready the passover.

And when the hour was come, he sat down, and the twelve apostles with him. And he said unto them, With desire I have desired to eat this passover with you before I suffer: For I say unto you, I will not any more eat thereof, until it be fulfilled in the kingdom of God.

And he took the cup, and gave thanks, and said, Take this, and divide it among yourselves: For I say unto you, I will not drink of the fruit of the vine, until the kingdom of God shall come.

And he took bread, and gave thanks, and brake it, and gave unto them, saying, This is my body which is given for you: this do in remembrance of me. Likewise also the cup after supper, saying, This cup is the new testament in my blood, which is shed for you.

But, behold, the hand of him that betrayeth me is with me on the table. And truly the Son of man goeth, as it was determined: but woe unto that man by whom he is betrayed! And they began to enquire among themselves, which of them it was that should do this thing.

Detail from The Passion, *1470–71 by Hans Memling. Image © Galleria Sabauda, Turin, Italy/Bridgeman Images*

The Arrest and Crucifixion

Mark 14:32–46; John 19:16b–18, 29–30

And they came to a place which was named Gethsemane: and he saith to his disciples, Sit ye here, while I shall pray. And he taketh with him Peter and James and John, and began to be sore amazed, and to be very heavy; And saith unto them, My soul is exceeding sorrowful unto death: tarry ye here, and watch. And he went forward a little, and fell on the ground, and prayed that, if it were possible, the hour might pass from him. And he said, Abba, Father, all things are possible unto thee; take away this cup from me: nevertheless not what I will, but what thou wilt.

And he cometh, and findeth them sleeping, and saith unto Peter, Simon, sleepest thou? couldest not thou watch one hour? Watch ye and pray, lest ye enter into temptation. The spirit truly is ready, but the flesh is weak. And again he went away, and prayed, and spake the same words.

And when he returned, he found them asleep again, (for their eyes were heavy,) neither wist they what to answer him. And he cometh the third time, and saith unto them, Sleep on now, and take your rest: it is enough, the hour is come; behold, the Son of man is betrayed into the hands of sinners. Rise up, let us go; lo, he that betrayeth me is at hand.

And immediately, while he yet spake, cometh Judas, one of the twelve, and with him a great multitude with swords and staves, from the chief priests and the scribes and the elders.

And he that betrayed him had given them a token, saying, Whomsoever I shall kiss, that same is he; take him, and lead him away safely. And as soon as he was come, he goeth straightway to him, and saith, Master, master; and kissed him.

And they laid their hands on him, and took him. . . .

And they took Jesus, and led him away. And he bearing his cross went forth into a place called the place of a skull, which is called in the Hebrew Golgotha: Where they crucified him, and two other with him, on either side one, and Jesus in the midst. . . .

Now there was set a vessel full of vinegar: and they filled a spunge with vinegar, and put it upon hyssop, and put it to his mouth.

When Jesus therefore had received the vinegar, he said, It is finished: and he bowed his head, and gave up the ghost.

Detail from THE PASSION, *1470–71 by Hans Memling. Image © Galleria Sabauda, Turin, Italy/Bridgeman Images*

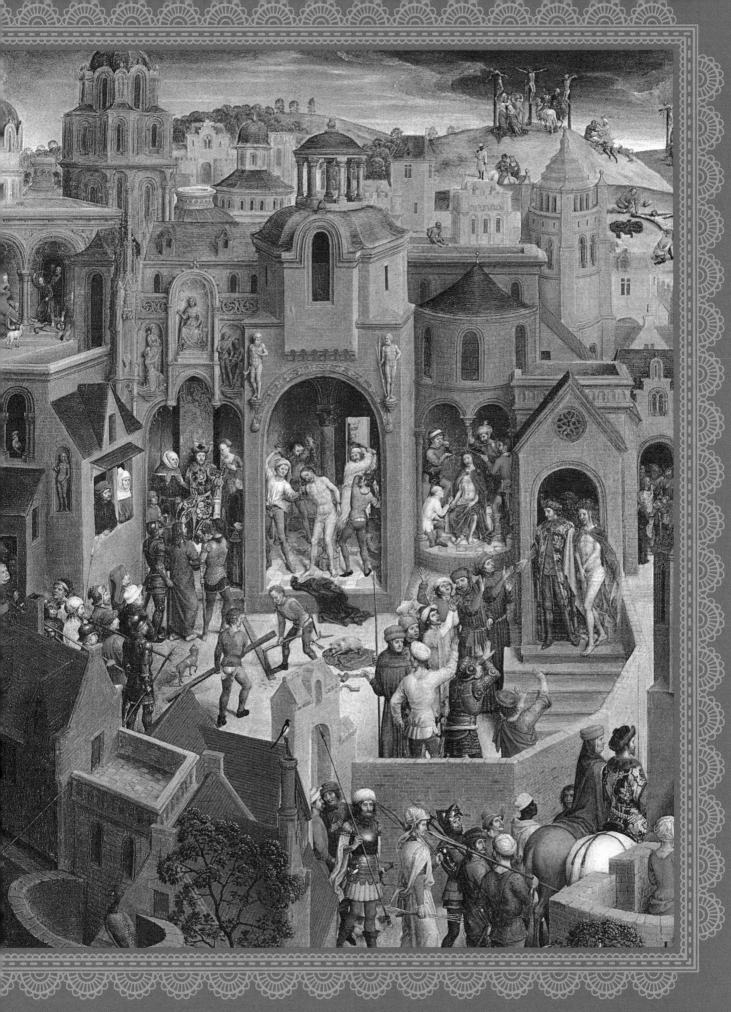

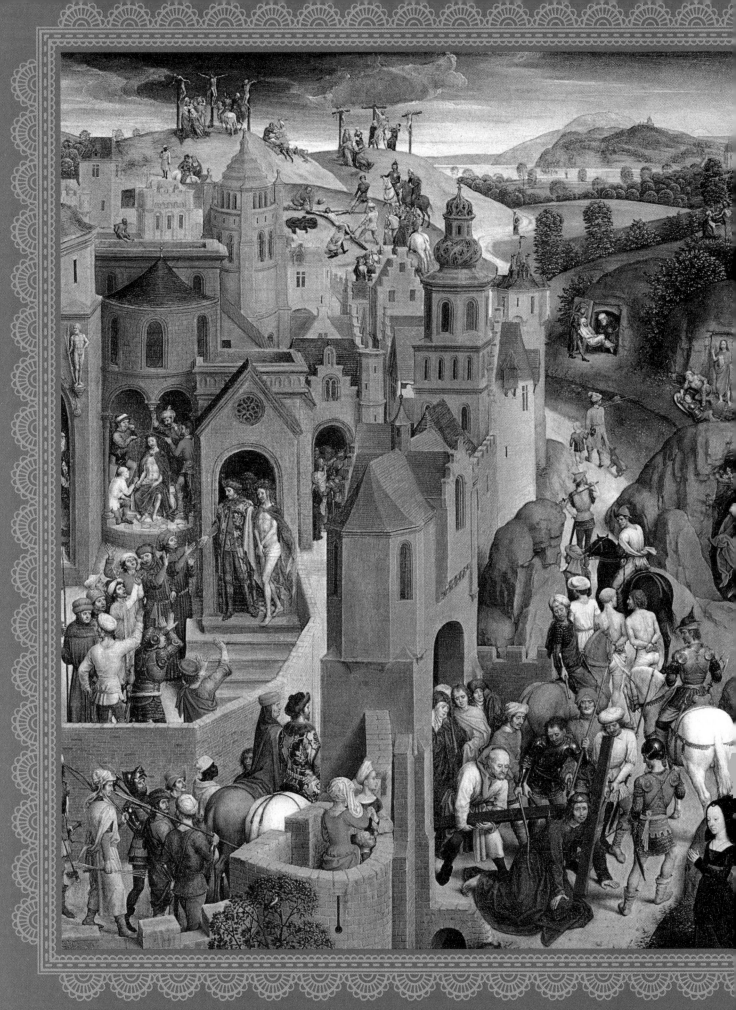

The Resurrection

John 20:1–18

The first day of the week cometh Mary Magdalene early, when it was yet dark, unto the sepulchre, and seeth the stone taken away from the sepulchre. Then she runneth, and cometh to Simon Peter, and to the other disciple, whom Jesus loved, and saith unto them, They have taken away the Lord out of the sepulchre, and we know not where they have laid him.

Peter therefore went forth, and that other disciple, and came to the sepulchre. So they ran both together: and the other disciple did outrun Peter, and came first to the sepulchre. And he stooping down, and looking in, saw the linen clothes lying; yet went he not in. Then cometh Simon Peter following him, and went into the sepulchre, and seeth the linen clothes lie, And the napkin, that was about his head, not lying with the linen clothes, but wrapped together in a place by itself. Then went in also that other disciple, which came first to the sepulchre, and he saw, and believed. For as yet they knew not the scripture, that he must rise again from the dead. Then the disciples went away again unto their own home.

But Mary stood without at the sepulchre weeping: and as she wept, she stooped down, and looked into the sepulchre, And seeth two angels in white sitting, the one at the head, and the other at the feet, where the body of Jesus had lain.

And they say unto her, Woman, why weepest thou?

She saith unto them, Because they have taken away my Lord, and I know not where they have laid him. And when she had thus said, she turned herself back, and saw Jesus standing, and knew not that it was Jesus.

Jesus saith unto her, Woman, why weepest thou? whom seekest thou?

She, supposing him to be the gardener, saith unto him, Sir, if thou have borne him hence, tell me where thou hast laid him, and I will take him away.

Jesus saith unto her, Mary.

She turned herself, and saith unto him, Rabboni; which is to say, Master.

Jesus saith unto her, Touch me not; for I am not yet ascended to my Father: but go to my brethren, and say unto them, I ascend unto my Father, and your Father; and to my God, and your God.

Mary Magdalene came and told the disciples that she had seen the Lord, and that he had spoken these things unto her.

Detail from THE PASSION, *1470–71 by Hans Memling. Image © Galleria Sabauda, Turin, Italy/Bridgeman Images*

Always Easter
Grace V. Watkins

You say it happened long ago
and in a far-off land
where men and women spoke a tongue
I would not understand,
that centuries have come and gone
since that triumphant day,
and that the garden where He walked
is half a world away.

He walks in every garden, friend;
and every rock-sealed tomb
opens 'neath His shining hand
as springtime flowers bloom.
For every dawn is Easter dawn:
on every sunrise hill
the earthbound glimpse eternity
and meet the Master still.

• • • •

In the bonds of death He lay who for our offense was slain;
but the Lord is risen today: Christ hath brought us life again.
Wherefore let us all rejoice, singing loud with cheerful voice—
Hallelujah!

—MARTIN LUTHER

• • • •

He Passed This Way
Letitia Morse Nash

He passed this way, and sleeping earth
springs to life beneath His feet;
the seeds and bulbs that dormant lay
send forth a message, green and sweet.
The hard, bare trees that for long months
gave not a sign of growth or life
burst into leaf and blossom fair,
and all the earth with joy is rife.
Tall Easter lilies, white and fair,
proclaim the triumph of our King.
He passed this way, and all the earth
shall joyously His praises sing.

He passed this way, and stumbling feet
walk straight and sure because He came.
And hands that faltered at their task
are blessed and strengthened in His name.
He makes the groping blind to see,
the deaf to hear, the dumb to speak,
and brings a blessing of sweet peace
to troubled ones that comfort seek.
He heals the broken hearts of men
and does their haunting fears allay.
And earth may hope this Eastertime
because our Savior passed this way.

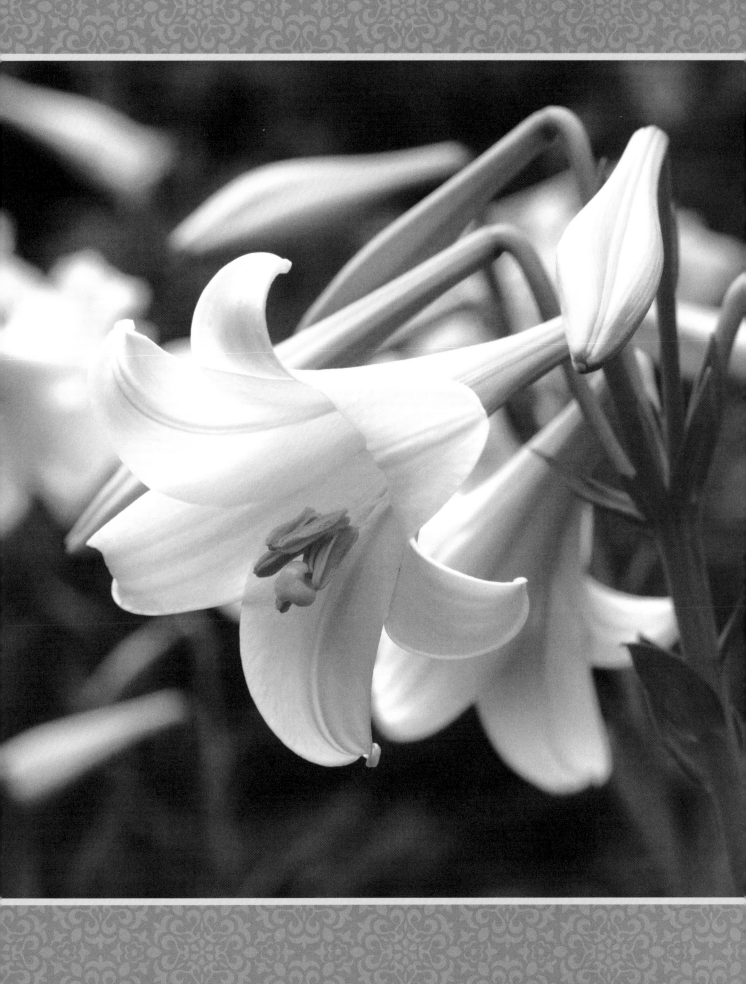

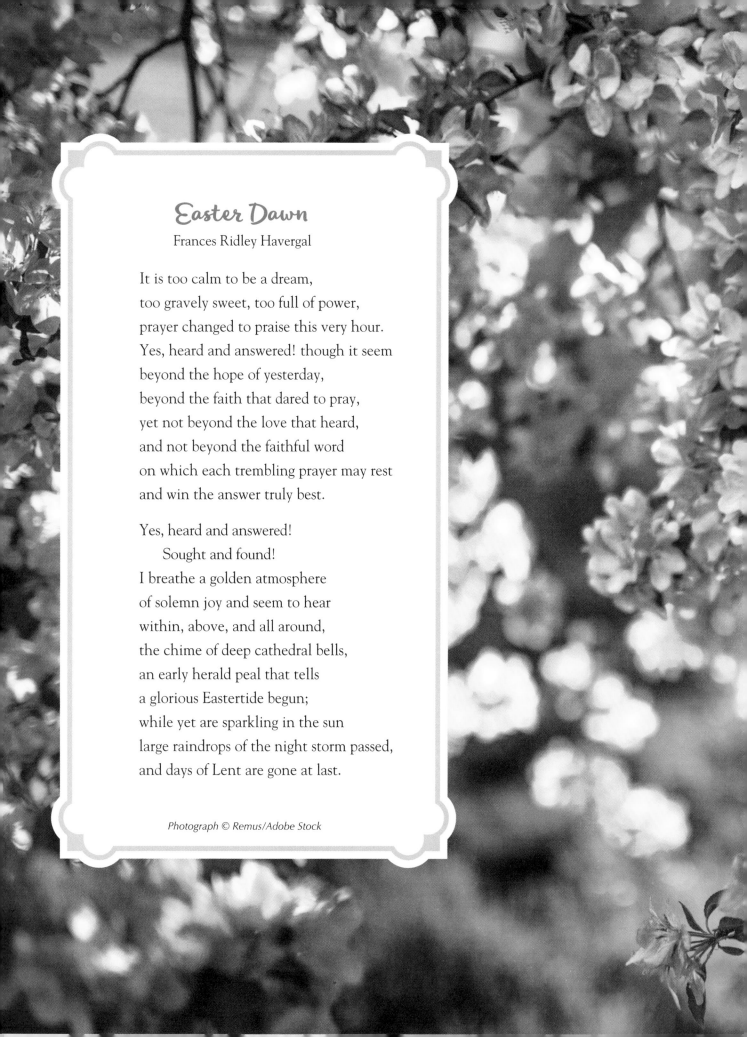

Easter Dawn

Frances Ridley Havergal

It is too calm to be a dream,
too gravely sweet, too full of power,
prayer changed to praise this very hour.
Yes, heard and answered! though it seem
beyond the hope of yesterday,
beyond the faith that dared to pray,
yet not beyond the love that heard,
and not beyond the faithful word
on which each trembling prayer may rest
and win the answer truly best.

Yes, heard and answered!
    Sought and found!
I breathe a golden atmosphere
of solemn joy and seem to hear
within, above, and all around,
the chime of deep cathedral bells,
an early herald peal that tells
a glorious Eastertide begun;
while yet are sparkling in the sun
large raindrops of the night storm passed,
and days of Lent are gone at last.

Photograph © Remus/Adobe Stock

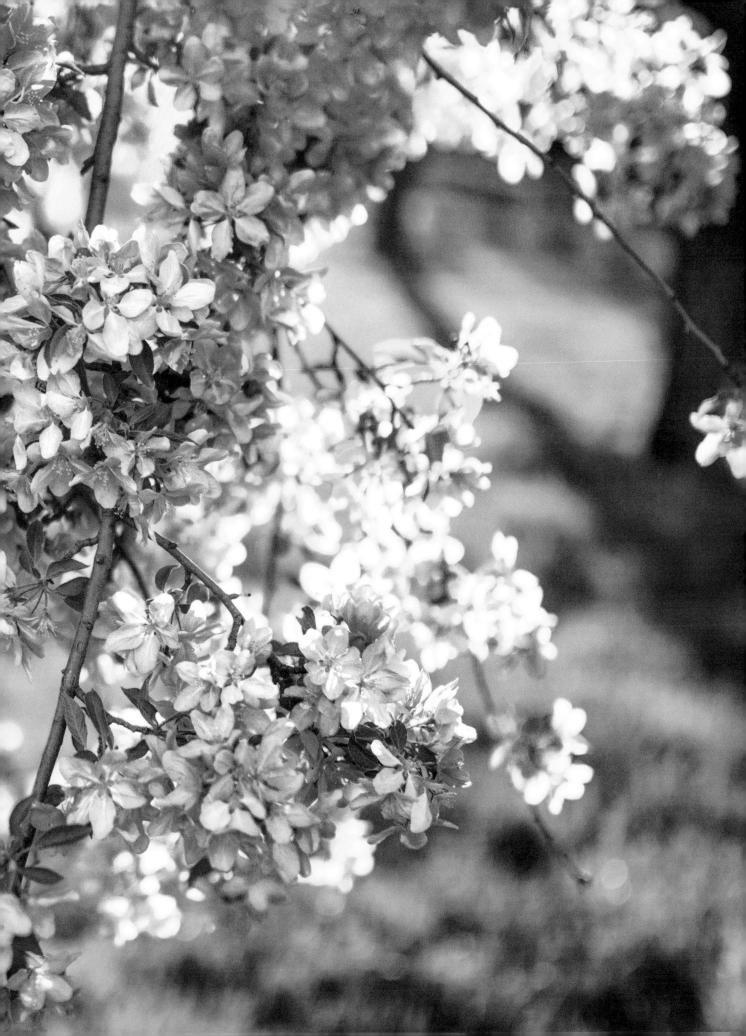

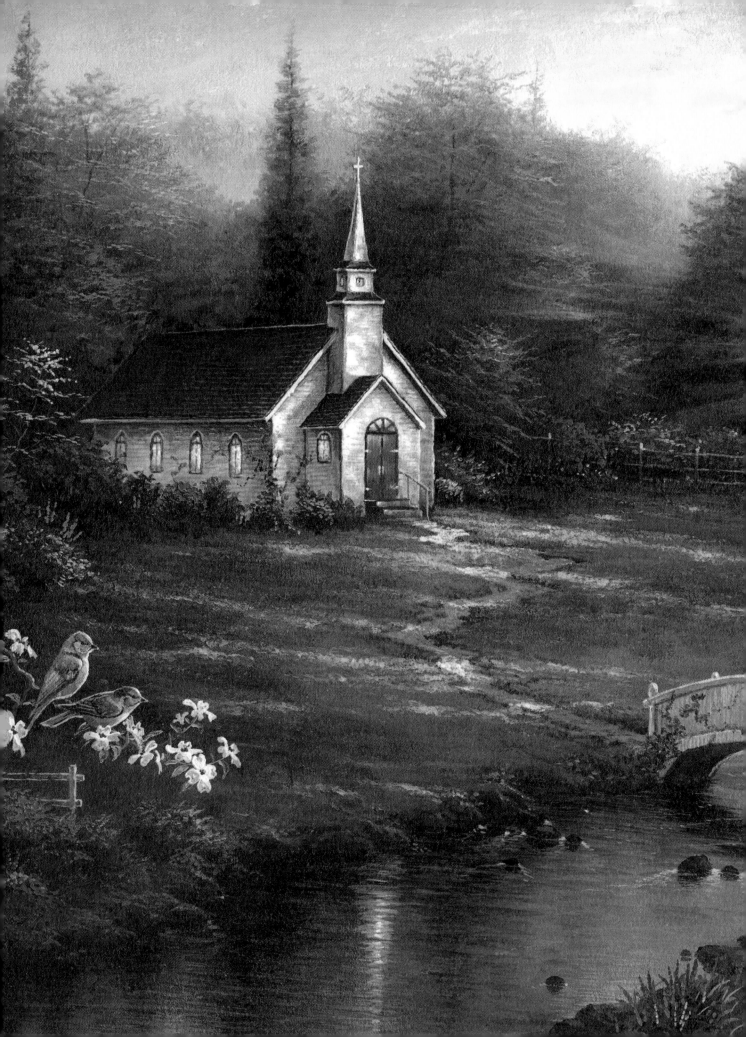

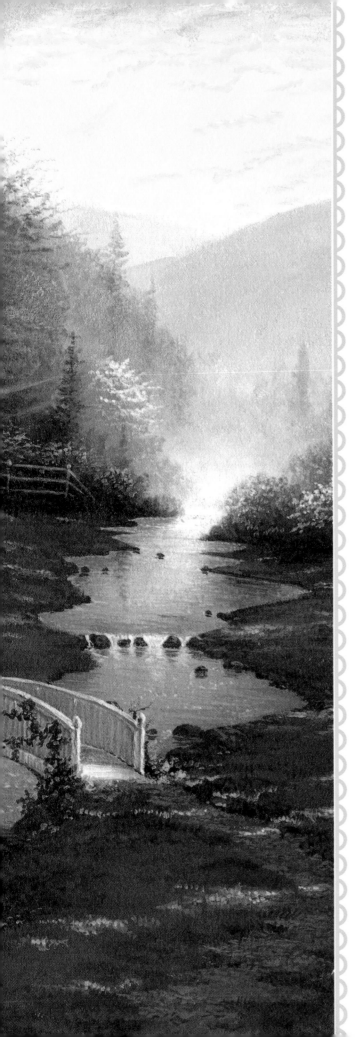

Tell It Well
Eva N. Ehrman

All dressed in our Sunday best,
some new, some old but clean
        and pressed,
we go to church. We hear its bell
calling us to sing and pray,
to give God thanks for Jesus' day,
for He is risen, it bids us tell—
He is risen! Tell it well!

The Church in the Valley
Loise Pinkerton Fritz

There's a little white church in the valley,
nearby where the still waters flow,
and where, in the beauty of springtime,
the colorful wildflowers grow.

A little white church with a steeple
in which hangs a golden-hued bell
that chimes out so sweetly each Sunday,
echoing all through the dell.

In this little white church in the valley,
theres's a special rejoicing today;
for here in the beauty of springtime,
Easter is holding full sway.

Its spirit sets heartstrings to singing
this message of newness and life,
a truth that will keep on blooming
when past is this Eastertide.

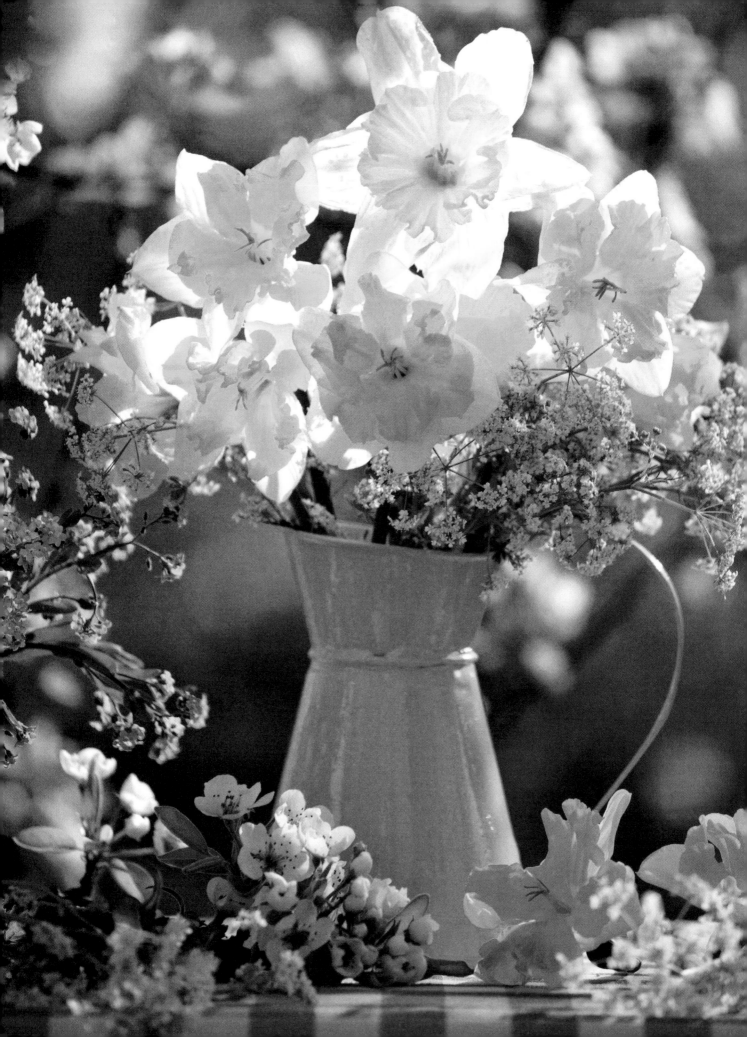

Easter
Johnielu Barber Bradford

Perhaps you looked upon the dawn
and saw the evidence of spring.
You may have walked where lilies bloom,
or heard an early robin sing;
or lovelier still, perhaps you caught
the first coral rays of eastern light.
Perhaps you stood upon a hill
and watched the sun come into sight.
Or did you wake on Easter morn
and turn your thoughts to Calvary?
Or did you see beyond the cross
a risen Christ . . . a victory!

The Heart Finds Hope
Virginia Katherine Oliver

The heart finds hope at Eastertime
and faith anew is born
as something rare and beautiful
on every Easter morn.

The soul looks up at
    Eastertime
while, humbly, men recall
the glory of a victory
the Master won for all.

Life means more at Eastertime
because on one glad day
a loving Savior
    conquered death
when He had passed this way.

Spring Hope
Lynda Schlomann

As we see the young grass
peep greenly through the earth;
as we hear the tiny birds
sing with bubbling mirth;

as we see the wild geese
return through the pathless sky,
honking over town and field
their triumphant gallant cry;

as we feel the fine spring rain
upon our upturned face;
as we see and love it all—
we feel Christ's embrace.

As the Easter sun is shining,
our hearts with hope will glow.
We feel hope and faith renewed—
for Christ has willed it so.

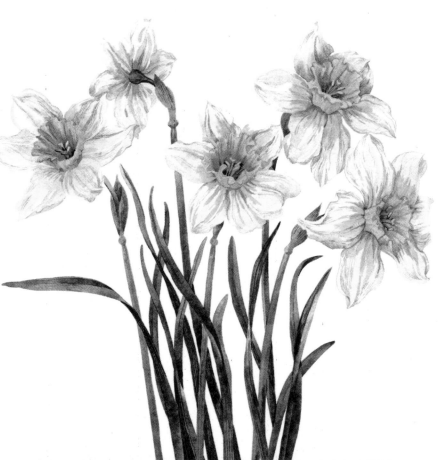

Photograph © GAP Photos/Robert Mabic

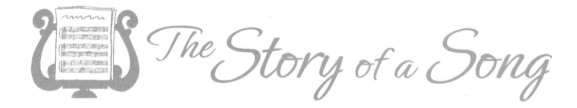

The Story of a Song

Shared Inspiration

Pamela Kennedy

Ray Palmer, born in Rhode Island, educated at Yale, teacher, writer, and pastor, might not be remembered by many beyond his immediate circle of friends and family were it not for a chance encounter on a Boston street in 1832. On that day Palmer ran into an old acquaintance, Lowell Mason. A prolific writer of melodies, Mason was in the middle of compiling a new hymnal and needed additional religious poems that he could set to music. As the two men chatted, Mason asked Palmer if he might have written anything that would be suitable for use as a hymn text. Palmer pulled a small leather-bound journal from his coat pocket and opened it to a well-worn page. He told Mason that, "The words for these stanzas were born out of my own soul with very little effort. I recall that I wrote the verses with tender emotion. . . . It is well remembered that when writing the last line, 'O bear me safe above, A ransomed soul!' the thought that the whole work of redemption and salvation was involved in those words, and suggested the theme of eternal praises; and this brought me to a degree of emotion that brought abundant tears."

After reading the poem from his friend's journal, Mason suggested they enter a nearby store where he begged a piece of paper from the clerk and quickly copied down Palmer's stanzas. He then declared, "Mr. Palmer, you may live many years and do a good many things, but I think you will be best known to posterity as the author of 'My Faith Looks Up to Thee.'"

Upon returning to his office, Lowell Mason composed a melody he titled "Olivet" as a setting for the four verses of Ray Palmer's poem. In 1833, the completed hymn was first published in a hymnal compiled by Mason and Thomas Hastings titled *Spiritual Songs for Social Worship*.

Ray Palmer would go on to achieve success as a minister of the gospel, a writer, and a translator of theological texts. He would compose more than one hundred hymn poems, but the prediction made by Mason would prove true. Palmer is remembered today mostly because of this one hymn, written from the need of his own heart, and shared with a fellow believer on a busy Boston street.

My Faith Looks Up to Thee

Words by Ray Palmer, melody by Lowell Mason

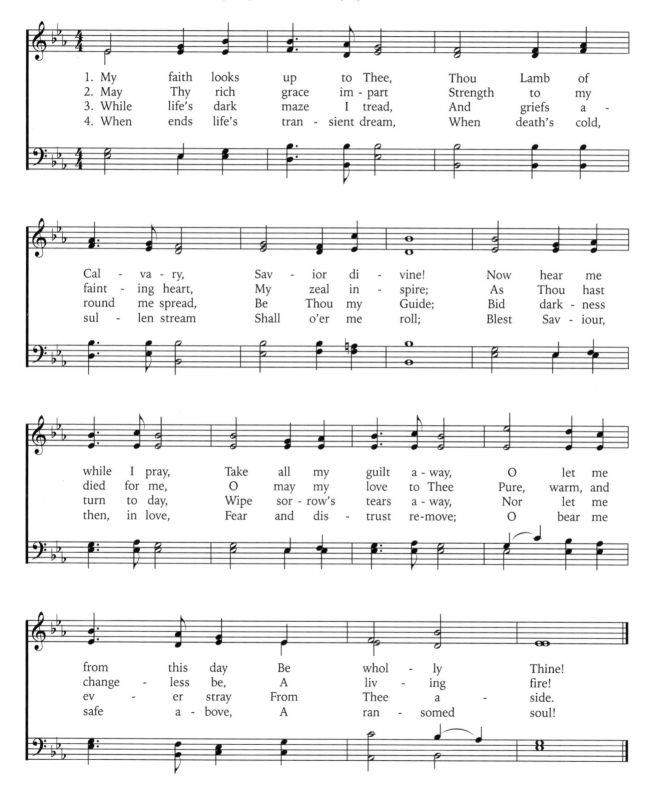

A Walk with a Child

Faith Andrews Bedford

My granddaughter, Carter, and I are going for a hike. I've loaded my backpack with some crackers, grapes, lemonade, and a diaper.

When Carter's father was a boy, we took many family hikes—through the rain forests of Washington State's Olympic Peninsula, up the White Mountains of New Hampshire, and among the valleys of the Blue Ridge Mountains. But it's been a long time since I took a hike with a two-year-old.

As we near the trail, my eyes take in the lovely woods, the colorful wildflowers, and the dramatic rock outcroppings. But we've a hike to do, so I don't dally. Carter leads the way with a little step that makes her look like a frisky colt—sort of a cross between a gallop and a skip.

Good, I think. *This is a fine pace. We'll make good time.*

Suddenly Carter hunkers down in the trail. "A stick, Gammy," she says, picking it up. She discovers another one and declares, "Two sticks." She places them in my hand for my inspection.

"Very pretty," I say, taking the little sticks and putting them in my pocket. Then I take her hand and lead her onward. "Here we go."

We walk hand in hand for two or three minutes until a flash of red catches Carter's eye. "Ooooo, pretty," she says and darts off the trail. Caught in the light of a sunbeam, a clump of car-dinal flowers glows brightly in the shadows of the forest. I follow and find her stroking the delicate red blossoms. She looks up at me tentatively.

"Pick it?" she asks.

I nod my head.

Carter solemnly picks one tiny bloom and lays it gently in my hand. "Is booful," she says, and I nod in agreement. I put it in my pocket with the sticks.

A few hundred feet further, we come upon a pile of boulders that fell from the cliffs high above. Of course they must be climbed.

As I hover behind Carter, hands ready to catch her, my mind drifts back thirty years as I remember watching her father climb the jun-gle gyms in New York City's Central Park.

We sit on a rock and share the crackers and lemonade. Carter gathers a few of the smaller stones and asks, "Pudit inna pocket?" I gladly oblige.

As we continue our hike (walk? amble?) I remember, too, that a walk with a child is about process, not completion. I slow down and let her set the pace.

By the side of the trail she spots a butterfly. I had not seen it. The butterfly is dead, its bright markings dulled, its wings tattered. Carter holds it tenderly in her hand and strokes its furry body. Together we marvel at the colors of its wings. She carefully picks it up and gives it to me. It joins the other treasures in my pocket.

A bit farther on, we see a line of ants marching across the trail. Carter is fascinated and flops down on the moist earth to inspect them. I lie down beside her. From this vantage point, the ants take on a whole new identity. They are not just tiny black spots but earnest workers on a mission.

I place a twig in the ants' path to see what they will do. Without missing a beat, they climb right over it. Carter fol-

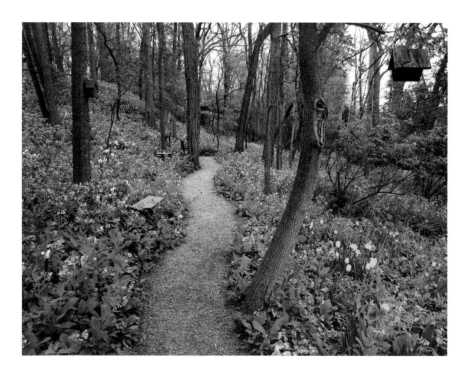

lows my lead and places a tiny pebble in a small break in the stream of ants. They climb over it too. We add ever bigger pebbles until finally we place one that is too large for the ants to climb. Their purposeful parade divides and flows around it.

Carter sits up slowly and rubs her eyes. "Go home now?" she asks. "See Mommy?" Ah yes, I remember. When one is sleepy, home is best.

For the past few months, whenever someone asked her age, Carter has been replying, "I pushin' two." Tomorrow is her birthday; we are visiting for the festivities. Part of my reason for this outing with Carter is so that Jill can put up decorations and bake the birthday cake.

We start back down the trail, more slowly this time. We've probably gone no more than a half mile. But my pockets are bulging and we've seen many new things.

I make a mental note that, next time, I shall tuck into my pack a magnifying glass and a small cushion for me to sit on while Carter digs holes in the dirt with a stick.

Carter begins to fret, so I move my pack to the front and swing her up on my back. A tired little head bobbles against my shoulder. As I slow my pace, I notice a patch of light green lichen with frilly edges. It looks like a crocheted pillow. In my powerwalk mode, I might have missed it.

To walk with a child, I have remembered, is not about "getting there." It is about discoveries, and rediscoveries.

"Thank you, Carter," I say softly.

"Tankooo," echoes a sleepy little voice.

The shadows lengthen on the path. In the distance I can see Carter's house. Birthday balloons are already bobbing brightly on the mailbox. Jill has put her afternoon to good use. Then again, so have I.

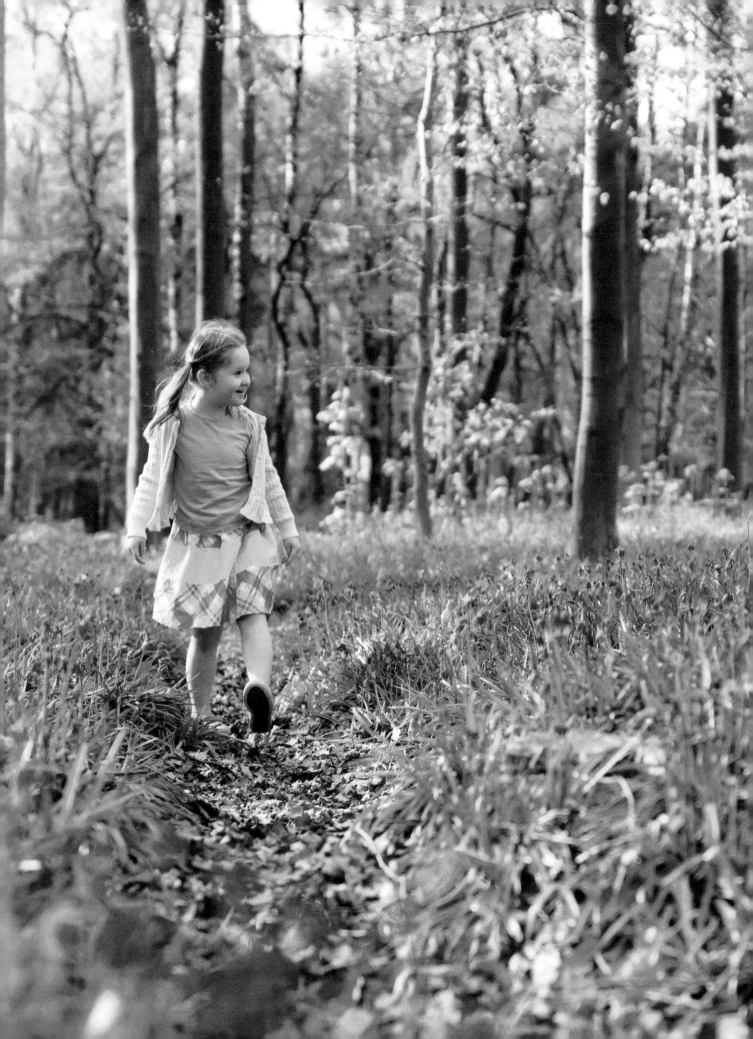

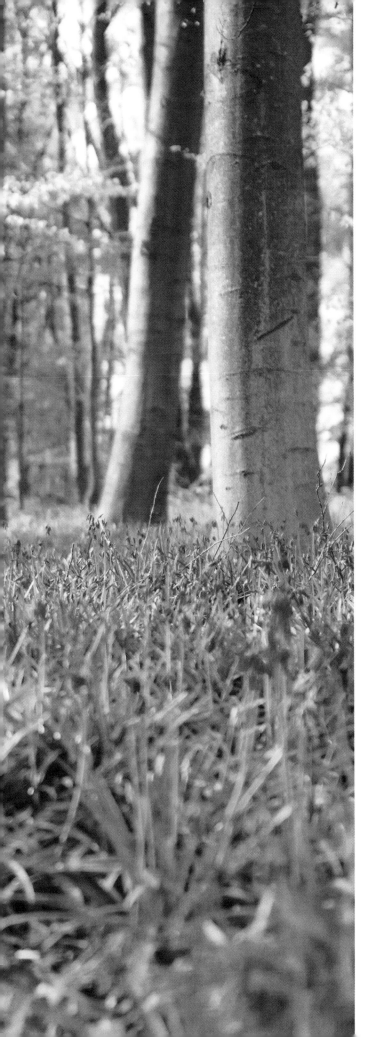

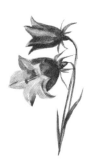

Prayer for a Child in Spring

Author Unknown

The soul of a child is the
 loveliest flower
that grows in the garden of God.
Its climb is from weakness to
 knowledge and power,
to the sky from the clay and the sod.

To beauty and sweetness it
 grows under care,
neglected, 'tis ragged and wild.
'Tis a plant that is tender,
 but wondrously rare—
the sweet, wistful soul of a child.

Be tender, O Gardener,
 and give it its share
of moisture, of warmth and of light,
and let it not lack for the
 painstaking care
to protect it from frost and from blight.

A glad day will come when its
 bloom shall unfold;
it will seem that an angel has smiled,
reflecting a beauty and
 sweetness untold
in the sensitive soul of a child.

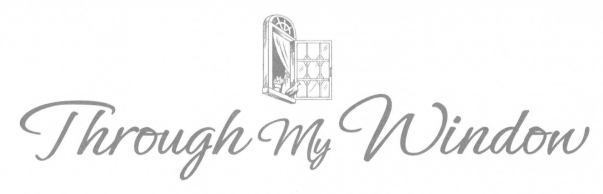

Through My Window

A Hyacinth for the Soul

Pamela Kennedy

I have never been much of a gardener. And moving from place to place every few years during my husband's twenty-eight-year Navy career didn't encourage putting down too many roots anyway. But I do love flowers. So when we retired and had more time to visit our family beach house near Puget Sound, I decided to put in some plants along the terraced bank. Lacking horticultural confidence, I enlisted the help of an eager young man named Mark who had a landscaping business curiously called "Full Throttle." I figured I needed someone with a positive attitude about gardening, and nothing says confidence like "Full Throttle."

Mark and I discussed flowers and trees and shrubbery and ground cover and eventually came up with a plan.

"Oh, and I want hyacinths." I added at the conclusion of our conversation. "There must be hyacinths."

When I was a girl, each spring my mother would purchase a potted hyacinth to bring home and set on our kitchen windowsill. The purple blossoms filled the room with fragrance and seemed to me to be the very essence of the season. We didn't have an abundance of cash, and these blooms weren't the least expensive;

but mother said it was important to treat yourself once in a while. As I grew older, every now and then I'd find a small gift in my room—a special hair ribbon, a new book, a frivolous bit of costume jewelry. "A hyacinth for the soul," my mother would say when I asked her about them.

When I was in college and, later, when I was newly married, Mother and I would sometimes go shopping together. If I'd find something that I wanted, but it was a bit of an extravagance, I'd look at her and we'd both smile like conspirators. "It could be a hyacinth!" she'd exclaim. She was one of the most practical women I knew— she canned vegetables, made her own jam, sewed most of my clothes, eschewed dinners out, and shopped the sales—but she also had a knack for nurturing our hearts with gifts of love. When I had a daughter of my own, I carried on this same tradition of bringing home a potted hyacinth in the spring and purchasing simple and sometimes frivolous gifts for her as "hyacinths for the soul." And we laughed about it just as her grandmother and I had.

I always believed my mother had made up our favorite expression, until the first Christmas after I turned fifty. That year she gave me a framed poem, beautifully rendered in calligraphy:

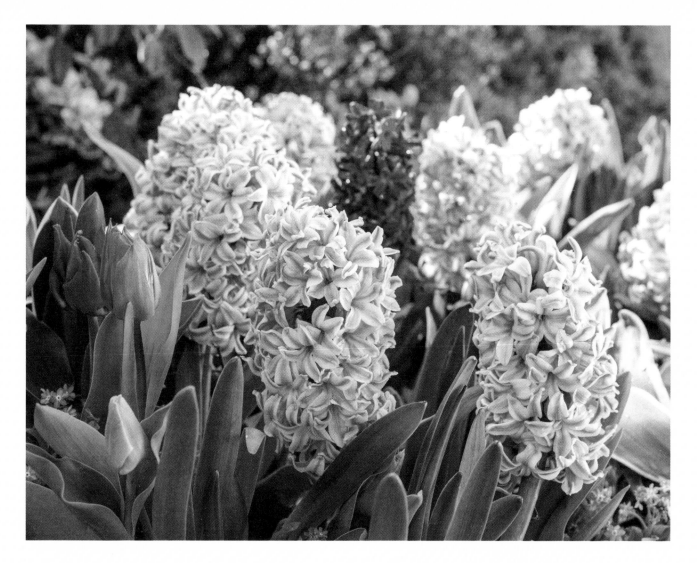

"If, of thy mortal goods, thou art bereft,
and from thy slender store two loaves
alone to thee are left,
sell one and from the dole,
buy hyacinths to feed the soul."
—Mosleh Eddin Saadi,
thirteenth-century Persian poet

She winked at me when I opened the gift, affirming this sweet lifelong connection between us and acknowledging that no matter how old I got, there should always be room for hyacinths. She taught me through this simple gift that nurturing the soul is just as important as nurturing the body. That love makes space for beauty.

Mother has been gone for a decade now but, as most mothers and daughters know, the bond between us lives on. Memories continue in the sounds and scents, the actions and emotions of everyday life.

That first spring after Mark of "Full Throttle" planted my garden, the creeping thyme ground cover tentatively made its way across the dark soil. Tiny leaves pushed themselves from the buds on the Japanese maple. The evergreen shrubs hunkered like wooly bears in their dark green needles. And in amongst them, my deep purple hyacinths stood like sentinels, proclaiming that spring was here once more and assuring me that my mother had been right all along.

Family Recipes

Sweet Potato Chips

1 large sweet potato, cleaned and trimmed
1 teaspoon olive oil
¼ teaspoon salt, or to taste
⅛ teaspoon ground pepper

Cut off ends of sweet potato and slice very thinly with mandoline. In a medium bowl, soak slices in cold water 10 minutes; dry thoroughly. In a medium bowl, toss with olive oil, salt, and pepper until potatoes are coated. Place in a single layer on microwave tray lined with parchment paper. Microwave on high power 3 to 4 minutes, checking often, until crispy but not browned. Repeat with remainder of potato slices. Serve immediately. Makes 2 to 3 servings.

Baked Chicken Bites

2 to 3 skinless, boneless chicken breasts
   (about 1 pound)
1 cup Italian seasoned bread crumbs
½ cup grated Parmesan cheese
1 teaspoon salt
1 teaspoon dried thyme
1 tablespoon dried basil
½ cup buttermilk
   Honey mustard sauce, ketchup, or
   other dipping sauce, optional

Preheat oven to 400°F. Cut chicken breasts into 1½-inch sized pieces. In a medium bowl, combine bread crumbs, Parmesan cheese, salt, thyme, and basil. In a small bowl, dip chicken pieces in buttermilk; then coat with breadcrumb mixture. Place on lightly greased cookie sheet in a single layer, and bake until chicken reaches a minimum internal temperature of 165°F, about 20 minutes, flipping halfway through cooking time. Serve with dipping sauce, if desired. Makes 4 to 6 servings.

Egg Salad Croissant Sandwiches

½ cup (4 ounces) cream cheese, softened
3 tablespoons mayonnaise
2 tablespoons finely chopped chives
½ teaspoon salt
¼ teaspoon pepper

6 eggs, hard-boiled
2 pieces cooked bacon, finely chopped
6 large croissants, sliced
1 cup spinach leaves, optional

In a small bowl, combine cream cheese, mayonnaise, chives, salt, and pepper. In a large bowl, use a pastry cutter or fork to mash eggs. Add bacon and cream cheese mixture; mix together well. Serve on croissants; add spinach, if desired. Makes 6 sandwiches.

Strawberry Pretzel Squares

2 cups crushed pretzels
1 cup plus 3 tablespoons granulated sugar, divided
¾ cup butter, melted
2 cups whipped topping
1 8-ounce package cream cheese, softened

2 3-ounce packages strawberry gelatin
2 16-ounce packages frozen sweetened sliced strawberries, thawed
Additional whipped topping and pretzels, optional

Preheat oven to 350°F. In a medium bowl, combine pretzels, butter, and 3 tablespoons sugar. Press into bottom of an ungreased 13- x 9-inch baking dish. Bake 10 minutes; cool completely on wire rack. In a medium bowl, beat whipped topping, cream cheese, and remaining 1 cup sugar until smooth. Spread over pretzel crust, covering crust edge to edge. Refrigerate until chilled.

Boil 2 cups water. In a large bowl, dissolve gelatin in boiling water; stir 2 minutes. Stir in strawberries; refrigerate until partially set, 1 to 2 hours.

Carefully spoon partially set gelatin over filling. Chill 4 to 6 hours or until firm.

Cut into squares. To serve, add a dollop of whipped topping and sprinkle crushed pretzels over top of each square, if desired. Makes 16 servings.

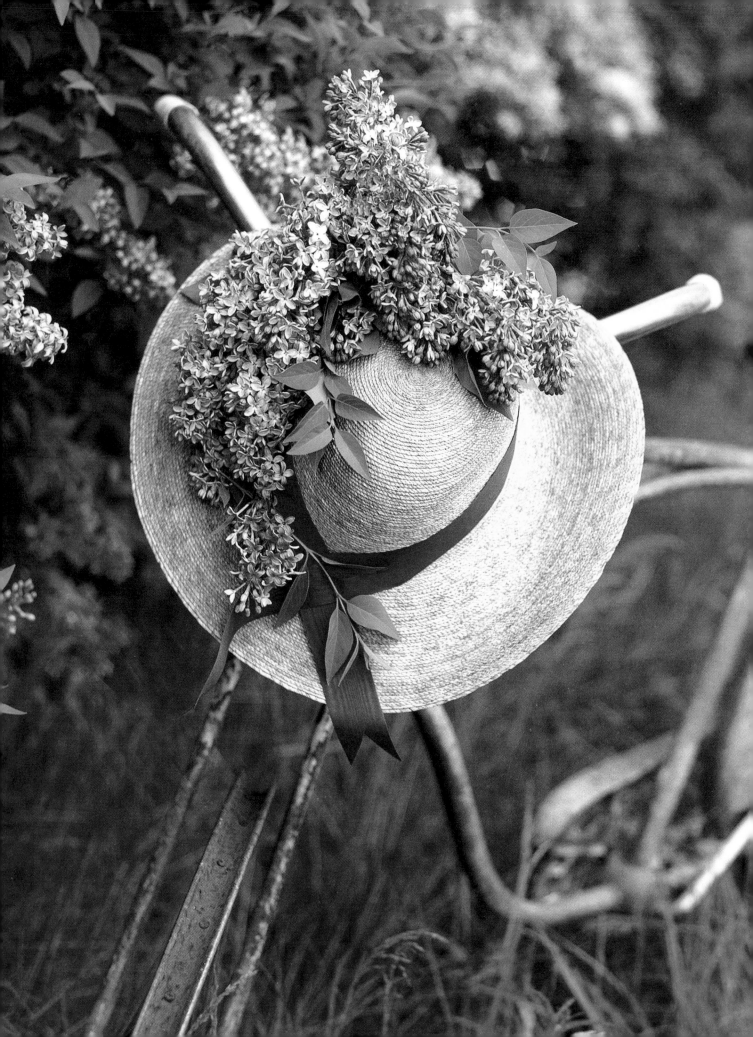

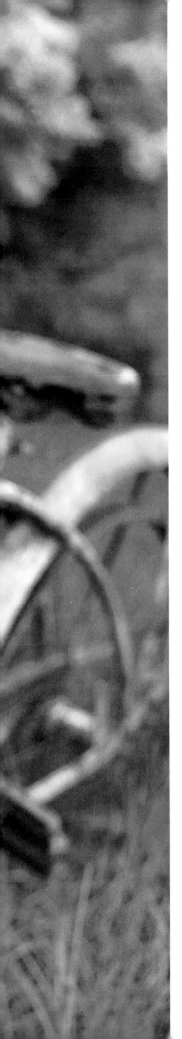

May Night
Sara Teasdale

The spring is fresh and fearless
and every leaf is new;
the world is brimmed with moonlight,
the lilac brimmed with dew.
Here in the moving shadows,
I catch my breath and sing—
my heart is fresh and fearless
and over-brimmed with spring.

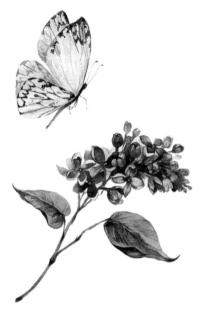

The Lilac's Fragrance
Geo. L. Ehrman

The lilacs are in bloom again.
Their fragrance greets the dawn
then touches every gypsy breeze
that dances on the lawn.
And then it comes in search of me,
no matter what I do,
to find a way into my heart
and set it dancing too!

Lilac Time
Brian F. King

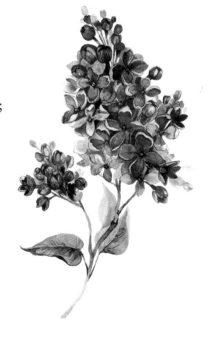

High in the hills is a lovely lane,
where sunbeams dance, where bluebirds sing;
where lilacs bright with gems of rain
wake to the kiss of the winds of spring.
Fragrant the scent of the sweet bouquets,
each purple bloom a fervent pray'r
that love will dwell in the hills of home
to bless each heart that is sheltered there.

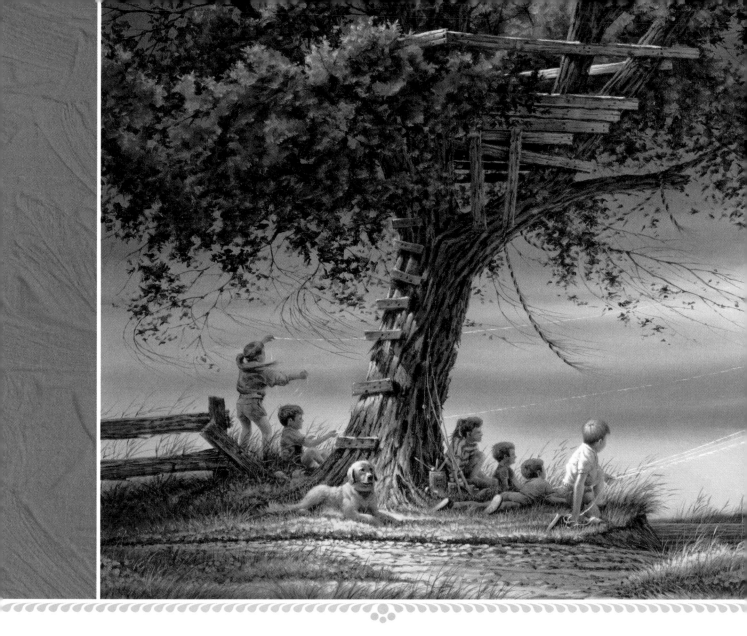

A Kite in the Blue
Joy Belle Burgess

Across the wide meadow
to the hill's farthest rim,
a little boy romped
with the frolicking wind,
with a kite that he treasured
and fashioned to fly
to reach for the faraway
blue of the sky!

Above the green grasses
and the buttercups' gold,
it danced with the wind
that embraced its white folds;
and it fluttered with grace
on its first lively fling,
as the happy lad grappled
and clung to the string.

Beyond the high treetops
and the crest of the hill,
the graceful white kite
was high-flying still,
when the little boy wished
that he could fly, too,
into the wonder and joy
of the faraway blue!

SPRING FEVER *by Terry Redlin. Artwork courtesy of C. A. Redlin, Redlin FLP, and Wild Wings (800-445-4833, www.wildwings.com)*

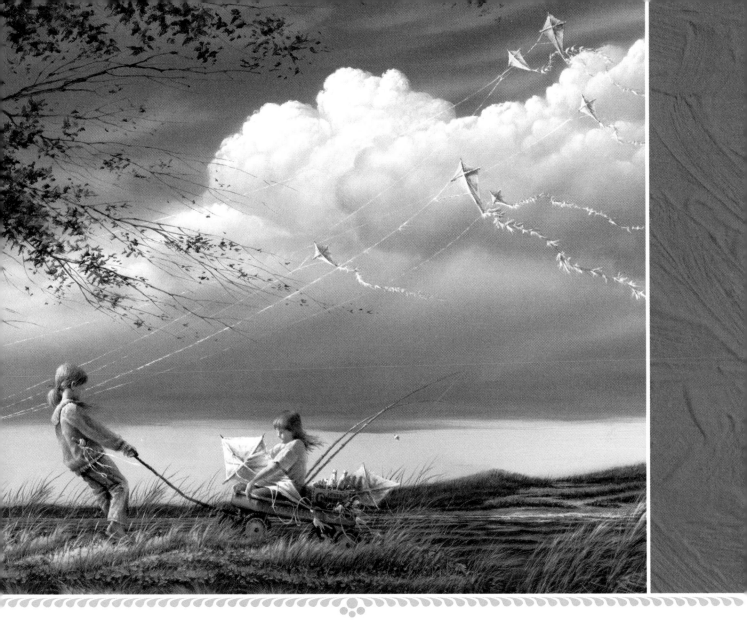

Definite Proof

Sheila Stinson

Rejoicing, I observed today
sure signs that spring is on its way:
a crocus skipped across the lawn,
ribbons of rose streamed from the dawn.

A small creek giggled with delight,
released at last from winter's night;
along its way the greening trees
shook their stiff branches in the breeze.

I heard two robins' placid talk,
perched side by side upon a stalk

of brown and withered bittersweet
(conferring on a safe retreat).

Just then came proof beyond a doubt—
a wild exultant boyish shout!

There, high above the tallest tree,
a kite in flaunting majesty
sailed by—its tail a thing of joy,
and at the string's end, breathless boy!
"Now how about that kite," he cried
and watched it with a boy's own pride.

My Mother's Garden
George Nicholas Rees

My mother hastened in the spring
to sow petunia beds.
She planted coxcomb, quick to bring
a host of feath'ry heads.
She sought to cherish every thing
that brightened old homesteads.
My mother liked to fuss a bit
about her favorite flowers.
Ofttimes she chose to sit and knit
through summer twilight hours;

she marked each moth
    that chanced to flit
around these fragrant bowers.
Her hollyhocks had giant stalks;
the cannas grew so tall;
primroses thrived along the walks;
shrubs hid the garden wall.
Her garden was the kind that talks
from early spring till fall.

Grandmother's Garden
Edith Roscoe Hilsinger

Grandmother's garden smelled
    of phlox,
forget-me-nots, and four-o'clocks.
Morning-glories, heavenly blue,
climbed the rustic fence to view
Grandmother and her shadow, me,
the little girl that used to be.
"Flowers talk," one day she said,
pausing by the pansy bed.

"Pansies are for thoughts, you see.
Roses, for love." Then, tenderly,
a sprig of lavender she plucked,
which in my pinafore she tucked.
"The sweetest flower of
    memory, this,"
said she. Then bent again to kiss
my cheek; and to this hour,
I see her face in every flower.

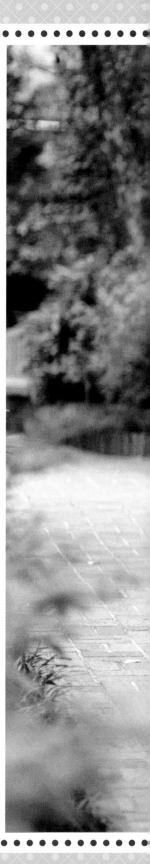

Photograph © danielsphoto/Shutterstock

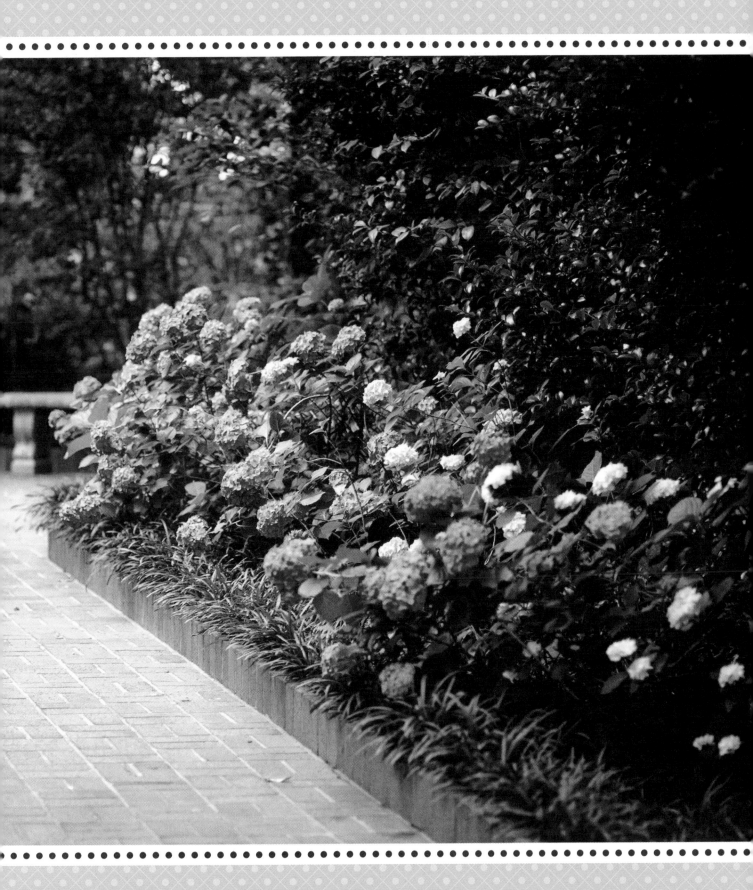

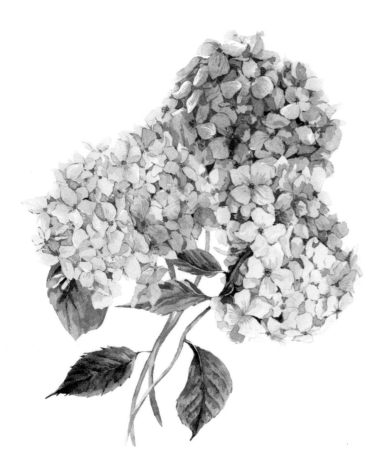

Springtime Fancy

Virginia Katherine Oliver

It may be just springtime fancy,
but it always seems to me
that in the spring the flowers sing,
and every leafy tree.

The songs of birds from every branch
seem just to lead the way
for all the earth to join in song
to greet each coming day.

It may be just springtime fancy,
but all nature seems to sing:
hail to this happy time of year,
the joyous time of spring.

ISBN-13: 978-0-8249-1353-3

Published by Ideals
An imprint of Worthy Publishing Group
A division of Worthy Media, Inc.
Nashville, Tennessee

Printed and bound in the U.S.A.
Printed on Weyerhauser Lynx. The paper used in this publication meets the minimum requirements of American National Standard for Information Sciences—Permanence of Paper for Printed Materials, ANSI Z39.48-1984.

Publisher, Peggy Schaefer
Editor, Melinda L. R. Rumbaugh
Designer, Marisa Jackson
Permissions and Research, Kristi Breeden
Copy Editor, Debra Wright

Cover: Image © GAP Photos/Friedrich Strauss
Inside front cover: Image © Depiano/Shutterstock.com
Inside back cover: Image © Depiano/Shutterstock.com
Additional art credits: Artwork for "Bits & Pieces," "Family Recipes, and "The Story of a Song" by Lisa Reed. Sheet music for "My Faith Looks Up to Thee" by Dick Torrans, Melode, Inc.

ACKNOWLEDGMENTS

BEDFORD, FAITH ANDREWS. "A Walk with a Child" from CountryLiving.com, May 1998. All rights reserved. Used by permission of the author. LA FERLE, CINDY. "A Fine-Feathered Easter" from *Writing Home* © 2005. Cindylaferlehappythings.blogspot.com. All rights reserved. Used by permission of the author. DR. RALPH F. WILSON. "Peter's Story" from Joyfulheart.com. All rights reserved. Used by permission. OUR THANKS to the following authors or their heirs: Caroline Henning Bair, Bea Bourgeois, Johnielu Barber Bradford, Anne Kennedy Brady, Amanda Meade Brewer, Joy Belle Burgess, Marion Doyle, Eva N. Ehrman, George L. Ehrman, Loise Pinkerton Fritz, Edith Roscoe Hilsinger, Reginald Holmes, Edna Jaques, Pamela Kennedy, Brian F. King, Minnie Klemme, Brenda Leigh, Andrew L. Luna, Peggy Mlcuch, Letitia Morse Nash, Virginia Katherine Oliver, George N. Rees, Shirley Sallay, Lynda Schlomann, Garnett Ann Schultz, Eileen Spinelli, Sheila Stinson, Grace V. Watkins, Agnes Finch Whitacre.

Scripture quotations are taken from King James Version (KJV).

Every effort has been made to establish ownership and use of each selection in this book. If contacted, the publisher will be pleased to rectify any inadvertent errors or omissions in subsequent editions.